A WARRIOR'S WORDS:

A JOURNEY THROUGH TRIPLE
NEGATIVE BREAST CANCER

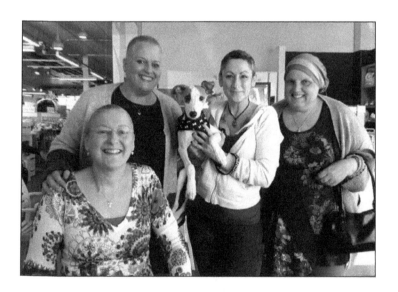

Edwina Maria Thompson

Grosvenor House
Publishing Limited

This book is published by
Grosvenor House Publishing Ltd
Link House
140 The Broadway, Tolworth, Surrey, KT6 7HT.
www.grosvenorhousepublishing.co.uk

A CIP record for this book
is available from the British Library

ISBN 978-1-78623-378-3

Foreword by Shine Bright Foundation

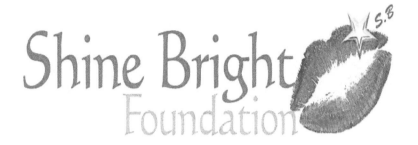

TOGETHER WE ARE STRONGER

SHINE BRIGHT FOUNDATION was launched in November 2013 in memory of Sarah Bennett. Sarah passed away in August 2013 aged 32 after suffering from Triple Negative Breast Cancer ("TNBC"). TNBC is a type of breast cancer, which unlike other types of breast cancer, does not have receptors for the hormones oestrogen and progesterone or the protein HER2 limiting the treatments available. TNBC affects more women under the age of 40.

It was Sarah's request that her family and friends establish a charity to raise money for research into TNBC and also to offer support to people in the local area affected by breast cancer. We are in contact with a leading oncologist Dr Sacha Howell at The Christie Hospital, Manchester who has a team researching TNBC and other breast cancers. In the 5 years since Shine Bright Foundation Charity began we have given £10,000 to Imperial College Hospital London for research and in May 2017 gave £17,000 to The Christie Hospital, Manchester to fund two new TNBC trials. Since that date and because of the kindness of people fundraising for us we have been able to give a further £30,000 to Dr Howell's research team at the Christie to continue to research to help find a cure for TNBC.

Locally in Cheshire we are able to provide 6 free reiki or reflexology sessions to anyone going through breast cancer. These treatments are carried out at the Navitas Centre, Crewe. In addition we are aware that people still need support after their treatments have finished. We fund an 8 week mindfulness course to help people to let go of the past, not to worry so much about the future and to live life to their fullest on a day to day basis.

Shine Bright Foundation relies on individuals and groups. Whether it's having a cake sale, nominating us as your chosen charity on Easy Fundraising, running marathons, or donating raffle prizes, every penny counts and we are always grateful to receive any help with ideas or any donations. If anyone is planning any events and feel able to take on Shine Bright as their chosen charity we would be very grateful to hear from you. If you know anyone who could benefit from our charity or would like to help then please contact us on any of the links below.

Facebook;   www.facebook.com/ShineBrightFoundationSBF
Email;   Shine-bright-foundation@mail.com
Website;   www.Shine-bright-foundation.org.uk

Shine Bright Foundation
Charity No: 1159185

WARTS AND ALL

Today, August 23rd 2018, is a pretty special day for me. Last year on this day, I had just completed 7 months of treatments for Triple Negative Breast Cancer. Back then, never in my wildest dreams, could I have imagined writing this Introduction. It amazes me that I am here now, doing this, writing a book! That is a lesson I've learnt consistently on this journey... that you never know what it will bring. Cancer, the treatments, the side effects, the aftermath, the highs and the lows; none of them can be predicted. Each and every one of us facing cancer experiences a different journey; even those of us with the same cancer. We are all so completely unique.

During this journey, my friends and loved ones have gone above and beyond, as they all rallied around to help me and lend their support. However, having cancer has also allowed me to meet many incredible women and men; friends have been made that I will cherish for the rest of my life. The capacity for compassion, empathy and kindness in people has both overwhelmed and humbled me throughout. Even through social media, people have been generous in giving of their time and their love: especially those going through cancer themselves and those of course, heartbroken to see loved ones suffer or pass away. I have known the best of people, at the worst times of their lives.

Due to my job as a yoga instructor, social media was already a 'platform' whereby my students, friends and family could be kept up to date with my classes. As my dear friend Wendy Austin calls them, my 'Tribe of Warriors'. I had, in a sense, been the 'leader' of this tribe for years. (Not a leader in my eyes though!) So after my diagnosis, this platform took on a new roll- keeping everyone informed of my progress through cancer. And when the call was sounded for help, the tribe gathered around me. From that moment on, they would always be there to protect and care for me; no matter what the outcome was.

At the very beginning, the writing was simply to tell people, day to day, what I was experiencing. Then, one day, an old friend Vannessa Taylor, suggested blogging my journey. (Another friend, Carol Ince, had been pushing me for years to write a book about my mad life and that was before cancer!) So I figured what the hell. Passing on lessons learned through yoga had been my forte for a long time, why not writing too? It came easily to me, writing; it seemed a natural progression for me to make. I was still practicing 'yoga'... only in a different form. (Yoga in truth is not about the impressive poses you see posted all over Instagram. It is so much more than that.) Then, as my journey developed and slowly the metamorphosis into the 'cancer patient' took place; out of the blue poetry emerged. Not a massive surprise as I had written a few in my past whilst training in India- but nothing on this scale.

My first poem was called Who Am I? And this was exactly how I felt. Who in god's name had I become now?! It was at one of my lowest points that creativity seemed to erupt. It poured from within me. I was desperate to show people how it felt to be this way: to not know who the hell you were anymore because everything that gave you your identity had gone. Waking up every day, to the cancer patient image in my mirror was debilitating. It was a whole new world of hell I was experiencing and the power lay in my hands, to let this be understood. I wanted to shout from the rooftops; look at us, look behind the mask you see; we are falling apart right before your eyes!

Once the flood gates had been opened, the poetry became my therapy. It was cathartic in every way it could be. It freed me from the thoughts, feelings and experiences I was embroiled in. It was my escape from it all. I could take cancer and turn it into honest, funny, silly, simple poems: turning Hell into a thing of rhyming words and fun. At first, my poems were only shared with my Triple Negative friends. These were a group of ladies I had met through Facebook; a group who were all facing down the same cancer: Triple Negative Breast Cancer. ('Triple Negative Warriors UK' became a huge support network for me and continues to be a place where anyone who is diagnosed with TN will always find love and advice. It is a fabulous group run by two ladies who have battled Triple Negative themselves- Carole-Anne Spicer and Colista Gaskin. Please, please do look to them for support if you are TN or know anyone who is.) Ironically, I was now a part of two tribes of Warriors- yoga and cancer; both of whom were there to hold your hands when you needed them. The inspiration for my poetry was coming from both my own journey, and from theirs.

As more and more ladies in the group asked if they could share my poems, the realisation dawned that they were truly speaking to them. In some way, my words said what others were thinking and feeling. It spurred me on, and for a short while, blogging became poetry. I would sit there for hours writing about my experiences; even going back to the beginning of my own journey, to turn my past thoughts and feelings into poetry. Sometimes, it would be something that I had seen or read that could set me off writing. My words weren't all fluffy language, hearts and flowers either, I said it as it was. They were raw, honest and brutal. But I also tried to be funny, hoping to make people laugh, not just cry. I wanted them to 'get it'. My poems probably shocked a few as there was no holds barred and I often had to warn my mother of what I'd written! (Yep, a warning to you too- there is swearing when it is appropriate and I say what others are often too polite to say!)

In my journey from Yoga Instructor, to Cancer Patient, to Poet; there was one special lady who inspired me more than anyone else: Julie Ainsworth. Julie and I had met through the Triple Negative Warriors UK group on Facebook, and were lucky enough to only live 9 miles apart. We would meet regularly at the local Garden Centres, or at her house and compare notes, treatments, side effects, problems and experiences about this whole thing. Initially, Julie was ahead of me in her treatments; but as her path took a different route, I became ahead of her. Where I had had a lumpectomy, Julie discovered she would need a mastectomy. Even early on, we could see that this 'Triple Negative' breast cancer was unpredictable and had no hard or fast rules to it. Soon, we were joined by another local warrior, Cath Quigley, and as we were both further ahead with treatment, we were able to support her as she too began her journey into the unknown. Cath would always refer to us as the 'Three Amigos'.

Julie touched me in more ways than I can begin to describe. I was blessed to have such a wonderful soul as a friend and warrior at my side through our journey. There was nothing we wouldn't and didn't discuss, and I am so lucky to still have our many conversations playing out in my head. Like me, Julie said it as it was, but was a lot braver than I in whom she said it to! Julie's journey took a more difficult and more tragic road, when she was diagnosed with metastatic breast cancer in November 2017. Yet she still managed to make a joke of it... "Only I could get breast cancer on my arse!" God, she made me laugh. As Julie faced down challenge after challenge, chemo after chemo; she inspired me by her incredible fight, bravery and ferocious love for her family. There are many poems in this book which have Julie's spirit imbedded in them, and they will remain in my heart and mind as a part of her forever. Julie truly was my muse as well as my friend.

This book has a purpose alongside the poetry, blogs, diary and insights of a cancer patient/yogini. It is also to raise awareness of *Triple Negative Breast Cancer* (TNBC). Until being diagnosed with this type of cancer, I had never even heard of it, but is a breast cancer that oncologists are working to understand. What they do know is: TN is usually aggressive, has a higher mortality rate, is more likely to return and that it tests negative for the receptors for oestrogen and progesterone and a protein called Her2 (hence the name Triple Negative). Therefore it can't be treated with the same drugs used to target these other types of breast cancer. Currently the most successful course of treatment is- surgery, chemotherapy and radiotherapy (as I had) and in most cases, I'm glad to say that TNBC is chemo sensitive. However that is not always the case. Since my treatment began, much research has been done; but on the other hand, there have been far too many losses from this aggressive and vicious disease. Quite simply, more money needs to go to research into it. This book will hopefully not only raise awareness for TNBC, but also funds into research through The Shine Bright Foundation. (I personally will be donating a percentage of funds from the sale of this book to Shine Bright).

This is my way of doing something for the many women who are facing this battle. I do this for everyone touched by TN, but also for my own family: daughters, sisters, brothers, nieces, nephews, cousins, for their children and their children's children. I hope and pray that this cruel disease never touches them.

My cancer journey has been wonderful, challenging, soul destroying, amusing, eye opening and life changing! I have opened my arms to every experience and there is nothing about my own personal journey that I would ever change. My blogs, diary and poems now take you on a journey through my cancer story, interspersed with Julie's. Let it be a celebration of life, love and undoubtedly tears I know, but with light and laughter in there too. May it always help to keep Julie's spirit alive.

Hopefully, it will continue to reach out to people and speak for everyone who has had their paths crossed by cancer. It has been one hell of a journey: and the most tortuous, heartbreaking but uplifting time of my life.

Namaste to you all,
Edwina Thompson

Warts and All

Well here I am, the other side,
A year has passed me by.
There's just so much I've learnt through this,
Now that I can't deny.

So many people there to thank,
From nurses through to friends,
Family, doctors, warriors,
My gratitude I send.

A 'poet laureate', I'm not.
I tell it 'warts and all.'
My poetry won't win awards,
It's just my messy sprawl.

But every word I write is true,
It comes from deep within.
They give a little insight to,
This path on which we've been.

For I am not the only one,
And yes, my journey's done.
But there are many on this path,
Forever must theirs run.

My poetry I hope will show,
The battles we endured.
The treatments, feelings, pains, the hopes...
That one day, Cancer's cured.

Edwina Maria Thompson
© 2018

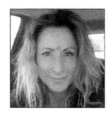

FOR JULIE

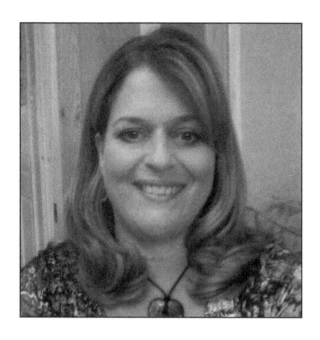

Now watching above, like stars in the night.
Her love and her laughter, so near.
Deep in our hearts, her whisper is soft.
Hold memories of me... right here.

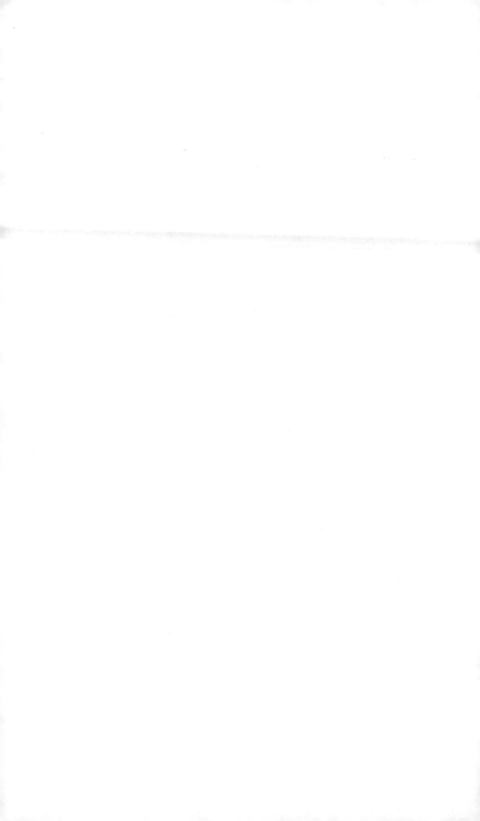

CONTENTS

A NEW PATH
TO TREAD

6th January 2017

Ok then, it would seem that my instincts last year were entirely correct; months of thinking something was wrong and there was. I have breast cancer. Not much more I know at the moment, I had no idea there are different types of breast cancer... so I wait. Surgery will be 23rd January, until then, I continue as normal. As normal as I've ever been anyway!

7th January 2017

It's funny how life can take such a huge turn, even when you sense something is coming. I might be one of the healthiest people going, a vegan diet, yoga every day, meditation, not too much alcohol (honest!), very little stress, and I still have cancer. I have had so many people say to me already... you are the last person on earth I would expect to get cancer! Well, maybe I am, but why? I am just as likely to have cancer as the next person. 1 in 2 they predict now, (in those of us born after 1960), will develop cancer in their lifetime. I had a 50/50 chance, the flip of a coin. Think about that, 1 in 2. Wow, that's a statistic to sit up and pay attention to!

One thing I do know is, never be scared and figure out what you're meant to be learning, and how you can help others through your own experiences. We aren't meant to 'get on with it' and do nothing else: we're meant to learn, grow, share, change, and evolve. I'm bloody lucky, I recognised a lump wasn't right and followed it up. I checked myself. Cancer doesn't need to be scary, but it is random. So, if nothing else... learn by my lesson, always, always check. You might find something, yes, but hopefully in time.

8th Jan 2017

So.... time to practise what I preach now I guess. That whole yogic 'santosha' thing: contentment regardless of what is going on around you. I've got it and I get it. I am kind of looking at Cancer in the face and saying- "Face, bothered!" (I do love Katherine Tate). John Lennon once said there are two motivating forces, fear and love. I chose love over fear, kindness over hatred, forgiveness over judgement. I chose my path, no one else. Never, ever be afraid...you will always lose. This is my 'dharma' (yogic duty) and I'm grasping it with both hands. Bring it on.

10th Jan 2017

Well, I have my official diagnosis. I have a breast cancer called Triple Negative Breast Cancer. I'm still getting to grips with what this actually means, but it would seem that the only course of action for it is surgery (with a sentinel node biopsy), chemotherapy and radiotherapy. How insane is that! The nurse explained everything to me, as I pretty much sat there stunned. As you can imagine, when she mentioned 'chemo-therapy', my first question was "Will I lose my hair?" And the response was "Yes". (Yep, I thought to myself, that's not hap-pening!) There is a thing called a cold cap I could use, but apparently you still will lose some of your hair and it adds hours to your treatments. Not to mention, it means sitting with a frozen cap on your head the whole time during treat-ments; and I've never been one for coping with cold!

Right now, I'm not planning on taking the chemotherapy. It just feels like an extreme option to me: but I guess I will seriously have to weigh up my options here. I have looked into it, and Triple Negative is rare, only in 15% of breast cancers. It also has higher recurrence rates and is more likely to spread into the rest of the body. The nurse has said treatments will last 7 months, like I said- I'm still working this all out in my head.

So, after this week I will be having my operation and easing my way back into teaching yoga afterwards. They will be removing some lymph nodes to check whether the cancer has begun to spread into my lymphatic system or not, (they will inject radio-active fluid into my nipple first to do this, ouch!).Therefore, I can't say how long I will be off work. I have realised I need to look after myself, and will do so. Provisionally I'm saying 2/3 weeks, but I've always been optimistic! I'm not scared, at all, but I am mindful of how those around me feel. Empathy is a powerful emotion and I must think of my family too. Regardless of anything, I will still always choose love over fear.

13th January 2017

Right then, I have 3 lumps, 2 that move about (benign) and 1 that doesn't (cancerous). I got the third one checked in April 2016 and was told not to worry, but do watch it to see if it changed. I only noticed the change in November I'll be honest. Yet, I knew all year something was wrong, my body was scream-ing it at me. Even lying in bed thinking, 'I've got cancer', fol-lowed by- 'don't be so bloody dramatic!' I had symptoms that wouldn't go away: a bad back, a sore hip in yoga, bad belly aches and swelling, weight loss, night sweats, you name it. Blood tests showed nothing, but it was there the whole time- cancer. It's true, it's knowledge you need, but also instinct. Listen to them, they will tell you if something is wrong. Simply put- know your body!

14th January 2017

In the last few days I've invited people (women!) to feel these lumps before they are removed. They are in appropriate places to 'cop a feel', but the difference with the cancerous one is very surprising. It is so small too. As was said to me yesterday,

'Oh my god, I would have ignored that, it feels like part of your rib!' Don't be frightened to ask, I would rather educate as many as I can. Oh, and no blokes, sorry!

24th January 2017

Thank you so much for your kind wishes, thoughts, love, chanting, chocolate, presents! I'm home and very sore, but that's expected eh? I'm very impressed that I should have 3 scars, very character building. I'll look like I've been in a sword fight, how cool is that! I gave them a laugh at the hospital too; after my injection of blue dye, I turned very green, and I'm the best they've seen apparently. The nurses called me 'Witchy Woo' and even brought other nurses to come and have a look at me! I'm still weeing green and that is freaky.

The whole process yesterday was a complete nightmare I'll be honest. I had to go to 3 different buildings before I had my surgery. Firstly, we drove 7 miles to the Breast cancer unit so they could draw on my skin where the lumps were for surgery. Secondly, we had to cross town to another hospital, to have the radioactive injection through my nipple. (This was so the dye would spread to my lymph nodes and a Geiger counter would be used to find them. The first few are then removed for biopsy testing). Thirdly, we drove back to the hospital (which is only around the corner from my flipping house), as this was where my surgery would take place. By the time we had reached here, my stress levels were through the roof; I'd had enough and just wanted the effing cancer out!

What astounded me more than anything though was the speed at which you are discharged from hospital. A lady opposite me came back from her operation at 2.30pm, as I went down for mine. By half 5 we were both eating our complimentary sandwiches and showing the nurses we were able to walk and go to the toilet. At half 6 we were on our way home, with a packet of paracetamol and codeine for pain relief. Unbelievably, she had had a mastectomy! They chop off your boob... and send you off home within hours. Crazy! It makes you realise how courageous women truly are. It also made me appreciate how incredible the NHS is, but how much it truly needs a lot more money to function.

30th January 2017

Today, I went for an appointment to have my surgery scars checked. I nearly fainted when I saw them! I know I was expecting to look like I'd been in a sword fight, but I wasn't quite prepared for the mess I saw. The nurse asked me how I'd gone on, and I mentioned how I'd been crippled with constipation. It had been so bad; I was eventually producing what looked like blue chalk. (Sorry about the image, the joys of cancer.) I'd been taking the codeine they prescribed me for pain, but had decided to check out the side effects. There it was, codeine causes constipation. As I explained all of this to my nurse, he laughed and said, 'Oh God yeah, that stuff will bung you up big time!' I am never, ever touching that bloody stuff again, I'd rather have the pain! He also told me my 'blue boob' is totally normal and that it will take about 6 months for it to fade. (That's from the radioactive injection) Wonderful, on top of the scars, I am now a Smurf too...

2nd February 2017 (A message to Triple Negative Warrior UK Group)

Thank-you for welcoming me to your group: I'm 47 years old, a yoga instructor and was diagnosed on the 6th January. I have 2 beautiful girls 21 and 22 and amazing support all around. I've had my lumpectomy last week and get results of lymph nodes tomorrow before anymore treatment begins. I think due to my job teaching yoga (possibly) and previous horrendous upheavals in my life, I seem to be taking this very calmly. Yes, I Googled, but took most things lightly, it's very easy to be scared by things, so I try not to be. I knew all last year something was very wrong, back and forth to doctors with so many different symptoms, my body screaming at me the left side was ill. Then, a small lump from April, supposedly harmless, grew. Glad I know now though! I love how this group is called Warriors, my favourite pose in yoga. My students call me a Warrior. We all are.

3rd February 2017

Results are back from my sentinel node biopsy, no cancer has been found in my lymph nodes! Way to go! Now to focus on my recovery, I may well be back teaching in a few weeks, you never know.

6th February 2017

Thought I would share what I'm trying to achieve at the moment, exercise wise. We sometimes think we're invincible and genuinely fail to appreciate how fragile our bodies can become. In my head, I'm a warrior, fighting strong and able to take on any battle ahead, full on. In reality, my body actually feels like it's not mine anymore. I'm learning to practice patience and acceptance with myself...remembering I have to learn to walk again, before I can ever run. The exercises I am doing are so simple but they knock me sick. All I have to do is raise my arm overhead or walk my hand up the wall and I'm not even close yet. Perseverance will hold though... I must give myself time.

15th February 2017

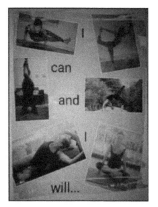

So, today I attempted a sun salutation (yes, just the one). I can safely say this does not appear to be 'my' body; it really is 'the' body. Every modification you can make and more, I had to do. No down dogs, no planks, no chance of reaching down to my toes, nothing I would usually do with ease. I accepted it, was glad of it. I was actually very proud that I got onto the floor and back up again, twice! Maybe, physically I'm not the warrior at the moment, but she is fighting her way out. She's in there, trust me, I can feel her. I have even made myself a folder for all of my letters, consent forms, treatments documents etc., for inspiration going into this journey. My new motto... 'I Can And I Will!'

17th February 2017

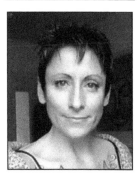

It's all done and dusted. My hair has now been cut short to raise Funds for Macmillan, and also in preparation for hair loss in case I take the chemotherapy route. (I am still weighing up my options here.) Meet the original warrior, the girl who fought her way out of severe depression and made me who I am today. If I had a patronus, she would be it! Don't mess with her, she doesn't take prisoners. Thank you to my longstanding hair dresser, Hayley Hodson, for resurrecting her!

18th February 2017

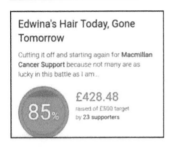

Edwina's Hair Today, Gone Tomorrow

Cutting it off and starting again for **Macmillan Cancer Support** because not many are as lucky in this battle as I am...

£428.48

85%

raised of £500 target by 23 supporters

Oh my God! This has totally made my day, and lifted me higher than I've been in months! This morning I woke up upset, drained physically, mentally and emotionally. I didn't even have the energy to cry. (Thank you to my wonderful friend Lynn Taylor for boosting me up again though; the lady who is in charge of my party girl and social well-being!)

But this has got me buzzing. Macmillan gave me £400 to help with expenses due to cancer, and so far you've all helped me give that back. I can't tell you how happy I am. I'd hoped to give back and give more if possible, so they can help someone else like me: thank you so much for making that happen!

21st February 2017

I'm now finally at a point where I have some structure and know exactly what is ahead for me. Next Wednesday I begin chemotherapy for my cancer, followed by radiotherapy. I've no doubt some of you will be surprised I'm taking this route; but after a month of thought, research, discussion, deliberation, meditation; I've made my choice. Don't for a second doubt that I know this is the right decision for me.

I am a mother first and foremost. I saw the reaction of my daughters when I said I didn't want to take the chemotherapy, purely because of what it might do to my body; and it was heart breaking. I cannot and will not refuse something that will help me. No matter how much yoga I do or spinach I consume, I have to do this! There is so much still to learn about Triple Negative Breast Cancer, and I am far from an expert. I must take the road which offers me the best chance of life in the long run. I will do everything in my power to be here for them, and always will. If the doctors said, "Cut off your arm and that will help", I would say... "Go ahead". I'm not daft though, I also have a ton of complimentary therapies alongside this! I am a fighter, and a mother... I know what I'm doing. My chemotherapy will last 18 weeks in total, 9 weeks spent on one drug called EC, 9 weeks on another called Paclitaxol. Yes, I will be ill, but I am young, healthy, strong, and fit enough to deal with it.

27th February 2017

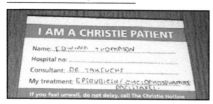

It all began to feel a lot more real today. I won't lie, being handed a card that says 'I am a Christie Patient', with your name on it does slap you in the face. Then a wig voucher to use (£63.35, how specific is that!) They also give you a booklet which takes you through your treatments; in it there is a chart of symptoms for you to monitor over the next 20 weeks of chemotherapy treatment. Oh, and then you're told you'll be learning how to inject yourself! You already know you are in this position, but now you're actually starting the journey...in reality.

I'm not scared; I am a fighter and will always be that. I believe we are only handed battles we are able to face, but I also believe we are meant to pass on what we learn from them. Life is short, and we live in a beautiful world we so often miss, because we are fed so much fear and uncertainty. We are often just too scared to take that leap of faith. Take that chance; make that decision, do it! As one on my favourite books says, F**k It!

THE RED DEATH
AND THE YEW TREE

1st March 2017

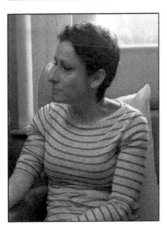

So today was my first chemo-therapy of EC (Epirubicin Cyclophosphamide). Actually, it wasn't as bad as I had thought it would be. (I wonder if I'll still be saying that in 3 months.) The worst part of it all was the insertion of the cannula. I have never been good with needles, and this was not a pleasant experience to sit there with it in for hours. This particular chemotherapy is red and after it has gone in, your wee turns pink for a few hours. Nice! (I've been calling this first chemo 'The Red Death' for entertainment value. When you fill in your consent forms, they list the side effects of EC... and it says death! Bloody fab I thought, I'm taking the Red Death, way to go.)

The actual room I have my chemo in, is lovely. There are big lounge chairs which are either purple or green, and there are beds there for patients who prefer to lie down. (Hee, hee, I'm looking forward to that day.) Volunteer ladies came around every so often with coffee, tea, water and sandwiches. It was like a picnic! I might add, my daughter had brought her own sandwiches and crisps, and did sit there scoffing away while I was shot up with drugs. I felt like I was the entertainment and she was enjoying the show, hmmm. On our way home, I did have a little nausea, but other than that I was fine. Not what I expected at all. We even stopped at Aldi to shop!

10

Yep, I'm keeping my fingers crossed it remains as easy as today has been.

4th March 2017

I was talking to my friend Vannessa from school yesterday. (I used to be a Primary School teacher in a past life). We've seen so much between us; it's been like a soap opera over the last 20 years. She suggested I write a blog. I'll be honest; I don't think I'd be much good, or funny; but I figured I could still write some of the thoughts I have on here.

A Mad Life

Sometimes I do look back and wonder; what on earth kind of journey is this I'm on? I've had a pretty mad, unconventional life so far. A very ill father from childhood (who taught me how to feed invisible animals that lived in our camellia tree); a boarding school by the sea (with 'afternoon tea' would you believe); the death of the first boy I ever loved at only 18; a university I never really wanted to go to, but still did. (I only went into teaching because all my family were teachers, and because some new computer programme suggested that it was my best career!) Growing up, if you could call it that, then meeting and marrying a man within 6 months- to have our first child only 6 months later. (Girls, I suggest you never do anything that I ever did...) Only a year later, going on to have another amazing daughter and getting a job at a wonderful school, where I got to work with many incredible teachers. It was also a place where I made many good friends and where life really began to move in an upwards direction, materialistically anyway.

At school we seemed to go through an unusual amount of trauma with deaths of a child, parents and staff; sometimes it genuinely felt like the world was a harsh place to live in.

Vannessa and I would often say it seemed like we were being given the same lesson over and again- that life is unpredictable. Yet at home, life was very different; we were just big kids most of the time. My then husband and I, along with our girls, had the best life early on. Parties, silliness, madness! I even remember all four of us tying our ankles together while we watched Children In Need one year, just for a laugh. (It became very amusing when one of us needed the loo!) It almost felt as if we'd won the lottery at times but in truth it was just sheer hard work from us both. We had begun married life in a small run down 1 bedroom flat with nothing and now here we were in a brand new 4 bedroomed house. There were trips to Lapland, Australia, Europe, Africa, all over- we really had such a blessed life. A life I don't think I truly appreciated and that was my downfall.

It was a pretty great marriage for a long time, with a husband who dressed up as Batman, Superman, Elvis, Starsky and Rocky Horror (on stage that one I might add!) I was Batgirl of course, and it goes without saying... we lived in the Bat Cave. Not even my married life was usual. Then it broke down, our own personal relationship devastatingly irreparable and completely unavoidable. Despite 15 years of marriage, a marriage that had been like a Fairy Tale at the beginning- it was all over. To be fair, both sides to blame in their own way, in hindsight. From there, the place I found myself in was hell on earth: severe depression is all consuming and it led me to an attempt at suicide.

How cruel can the brain be to make you actually believe your own children would be better without you? I reached a point where I could see no way out, with no light in the tunnel of darkness I was in. All I could see was the pain I was causing the ones I loved the most. In the broken mental state I was in, I believed I was doing the best thing for my children- by removing the cause of their dysfunctional lives.

I was no longer their mother, she was long gone. I had lost all sense of self-worth, I didn't even believe I was worthy of life. So one night, I took every pill I had, anti-depressants and sleeping pills. I got into bed and closed my eyes, ready to leave them all in peace.

Then something incredible happened... my youngest daughter came to me. (She had always been so like me we clashed a lot, which caused many arguements.) She walked into the bedroom and stood in the doorway watching me. Then she asked me if I wanted a glass of water, (unbelievable for her at the time). She brought me a glass of water, and climbed into bed with me. She told me how she had turned off the television and sky box downstairs, locked the doors and shut the windows. Then she said to me, 'I've made us safe'. I will never ever forget that, she was taking care of us all. What should have been my job. I remember very little of the next day. I know my girls phoned my ex-husband to come around and that my body and face was swollen the following morning, but that was the only result of an overdose. I have no idea why I lived; I certainly took everything I had. It clearly wasn't my time to die.

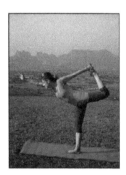 To this day, I think it was my daughter sent in some way to save me, crazy though that may sound. So my maternal instinct would kick in, and I would fight to stay alive. I survived and every day I have lived since, has been a gift: a gift that I cherish now with every ounce of my being.

I think that's the point I changed, I began to fight for myself. I found yoga of course and learned so much of life and love in the process. I went to India, trained as an instructor and thank God, discovered I could help untold amounts of people.

My own experiences seemed to help me empathise with my students, and for some bloody mad reason: they seemed to actually want to listen to me. What the hell?! This was a real turn up for the books; maybe I had something to pass on from this mad life after all...

Now here I am, on yet another path of my journey. Not once have I said, why me? Why would that even cross my mind? It's all happening perfectly. It's meant to be this way, of that I'm absolutely sure. Am I meant to pass on what I'm learning? I think so. I've spent the last 6 years of my life preaching the lessons of yoga, and now it's like I've been given a huge challenge- OK, clever clogs, practice what you preach then!

So what am I learning right now...love, patience, kindness, non-judgement? I think I was pretty good with the kindness and love; but I hold my hands up, the other two not so good. In fact I was pretty crap to be fair. I'm on this path, it's my journey and not everyone will understand my lessons or my choices. This is how we need to see others; we are not in other people's shoes. How can we possibly understand their path, it's theirs. Would I have ever imagined I would choose to be on chemotherapy? Never! But here I am, and so far, I'm fine.

I'm taking each of my lessons as they come, and one thing I do know, the moment I think I've nothing left to learn... I've failed in my life miserably. And so I continue to learn, every day. How incredibly amazing is this life, don't you absolutely love it!

11th March 2017

Well, this morning I got the expected from an older lady I know. Usually I can get away before she nabs me for a

14

conversation (I'm not feeling the small chat at the moment), but today I failed miserably to avoid her. Even after faffing in the car for 5 minutes before getting out, in the desperate hope she'd go. (Normally, I'm happy to chat but my patience is not as it was.) But no, she was clearly going nowhere, like a cat waiting to pounce on it's prey.

I relented, got out the car and accepted my words of wisdom for this morning. This was the gem for today… "My niece was young like you when she got breast cancer." (Oh here we go I thought, I know where this is going.) "She found out in the April, got married in the summer and was dead by November." Oh my God, why oh why do the older generation often insist on sharing their doom and gloom stories? You just have to accept them don't you? (What was that I was saying about non-judgement…?) Maybe in their heads, they are being empathetic? In which case, they'll never learn to keep their mouths shut I guess.

15th March 2017

A beautiful young girl so inspired me tonight. Earlier, I began to lose quite a significant amount of hair (not from where you're thinking though!) Knowing what was coming next and shocked even though I was expecting it, I turned to YouTube. I was looking for reassurance that I could do this and was led to Charlotte. She had uploaded a video on hair loss and I was really moved by her honesty and wish to help others. I decided to thank her and leave a comment. In doing so, I scrolled to the last comment to add mine… but it said "God has you now." I was completely stunned, and so went to her channel to see if this was true. Of course it was. This girl, so young, and having spent years helping others through this social media, had died. If you ever have the chance, please look up her channel, she is called Charlotte Eads.

17th March 2017

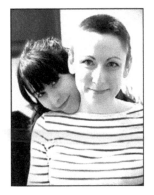

I am highly amused by my hair today. Ever since I began to show signs of hair loss, I've done the tug test on my head. (It has been cut shorter still now, a buzz cut which actually looks quite cool!) So far, it has been fine and holding on well. Then today, I had another go using tweezers so I only got the odd one and didn't create any bald patches. It failed the test miserably and the hair just slid out effortlessly, like nothing was even holding it on. And yet it's still there, clinging onto my scalp. How mental is that? So it would seem; my fighting/warrior spirit even goes right down to my roots. It reminded me of Independence Day the movie, as the President inspires the people as they go into battle against the aliens... "We will not go quietly into the night; we will not vanish without a fight!" Yep, that's my hair.

20th March 2017

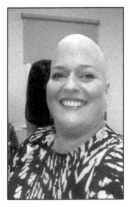

Today I got to spend the day with Julie Ainsworth at a Look Good Feel Better event run by Macmillan. Julie and I met up a few weeks back through the Triple Negative Warrior UK group on Facebook. It was so funny with our first get together, both of us peering at each other trying to decide whether we were the right person. When you wear wigs, you can look completely different to your profile picture! Julie had a wig that was quite similar to mine too. There are different types you can get and as Julie says, some look like a birds nest on the top. From a distance you would never know, up close you can tell. We are both already experts on the wig, and can spot one a mile off!

Today we were learning how to put make up on, ready for the loss of eyebrows and eyelashes. It's a freebee workshop organised by Macmillan and Boots together. I have this really bad habit of pulling mascara off my eyelashes with a wipe, instead of using make up remover; and you should have seen Julie's face! She was horrified and half expected all of my lashes to come out. They didn't, but bloody good point Julie... I best not tempt fate eh! It was quite funny at the end though. We'd been told you receive loads of freebies, so we were both waiting with baited breath for these fab goodies (£100 pounds worth we'd been told by some ladies!) Sod's Law, they must have been running low because all we got was a blush stick and a sample pot of foundation. It serves us right for expecting something for nothing I suppose, but we were still grateful though, honest! Then we went onto have a meal and coffee at the local Garden Centre. It's so lovely to meet with other ladies in similar situations. We got to compare notes on treatments and side effects. How lucky are we to live so close. This is a friendship I'm going to cherish so much. What a fantastic day, thank you Julie!

23rd March 2017

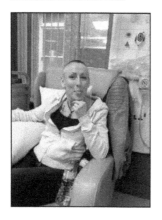

Last photo of me looking half decent with my own hair, I couldn't resist pulling tongues. It's being shaved bald tomorrow. Having my second chemo yesterday was a lot harder than the first. My body knew what was coming and reacted accordingly, it didn't even like the cannula! I felt every drop and the needle was so painful, I felt sick the entire time. Not being able to manage the stairs on my own last night was a real shock too and phoning the Christie Hotline for advice on how many drugs I could shove in my system was a first! Then lying in bed thinking is this what dying feels like? Today has been spent in bed, focusing on good things. Rest and recuperation is essential for everyone. Never ever take your health for granted, you just never know!

24th March 2017

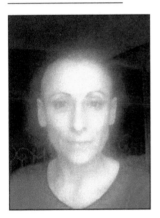

OK, so today I went the whole hog and had my hair shaved off. It had to be done. After the deed had been done, I gathered all my courage to go and look in the mirror. In my dreams, I envisaged Demi Moore in GI Jane smiling back at me, in reality I figured it was going to be more like Uncle bloody Fester from the Adams Family. (If you don't know who I mean, Google him). I gathered myself and looked. Yeah, as you can guess, I wasn't far wrong... a mix of Uncle Fester, Renton from Trainspotting and if I squinted, a tiny bit of Demi! Oh well, what the hell I figured, a fair bit of make-up and I'll rock the look!

My ego shot through the roof... my fire, drive, determination, will power, warrior strength, spirit, fight, you name it: it was there! I can do this, I bloody know I can. NOTHING can keep me down, ever! You know what I thought; I'll take a photo and put it on my blog. If I can present myself completely bare faced and as a skin head, I really can handle anything. So, I did it. I took the photo.... and look what happened. It's not the light, the sun wasn't even shining brightly and I've taken many photos in this same place. This has never, ever happened before. Believe what you want, but for that split second I think my aura radiated exactly how I felt, a true warrior. My Manipura chakra, way to go, you really do rock!

27th March 2017

Burst That Bubble

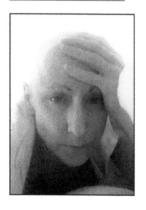

Have you ever just had one of those days? I know I haven't really allowed any of you all to see the crap side to cancer treatment. (Hence, I give you a dreadful pic of me this morning.) I've posted tons of pictures of me looking happy and healthy on the whole; almost as if this whole 'cancer' thing isn't as difficult as you'd think. It's me of course, trying to put out that positive light on a horrible situation. Don't get me wrong, 99% of the time, I genuinely feel that way, positive (and still do). Then a crap day hits out of the blue.

I'd be lying if I said this is easy, it isn't. It's shit, really shit (excuse the French!) I'm on a cocktail of drugs that have an awful effect on my body. Today I've been ill all day. (In between, covering myself in make-up when the wig guy arrived, and totally pretending I feel fine. We're British, it's what we do!)

I'll not go into details, but the drugs affect my stomach badly and today I lost half a stone in 3 hours. (No it's not a new diet plan, don't bloody try it!) Every day after chemo for 7 days, I have to inject myself with a white blood cell boost. Last time, I wasn't too bad; this time, I was useless. I've cocked it up so many times now; bruised myself badly, and given myself an even bigger fear of needles. I'm also frightened of meeting people who are ill as my white blood cell count has halved, meaning I'm susceptible to anything. And now I'm currently

19

lying in bed, writing this and thinking to myself, you've bloody waffled again.... what was the point you were making?

Yeah, I've been ill all day, so what, I knew that would happen. Mucking about with Senokot Max served me right! Am I after sympathy? Am I hell as like! I'm just being honest; please don't look and think, God cancer's not that bad is it. For me it isn't so far, but for so many others, it's hell on earth. Yet it's not just cancer that can place us in Hell is it? (And so we get to my point, about flipping time.) I get to lie here and think: how lucky I am. I'm not rushing around, letting day to day life and stress take over me. I know the difficulties many of my beautiful friends are facing right now, and my heart goes out to so many of them.

When was the last time you stopped, burst out of your own little bubble for a moment? Remembered that friend who might just need that text, a few words, a phone call saying, "I haven't forgotten you, I am thinking of you." We rush around in this world; and get so wrapped up in our own bubbles. It's not me that needs you today, it's someone else. Send them that message...break that bubble. Do it now, please, not in five minutes. Yours might be the first kindness they've been shown today; in a week; even in months. Today let them know you care.

3rd April 2017

I am, I think, finally ready to roll out my mat tonight and go to a class. (Rather than the 10 minute mini yoga poses I've been doing.). I am part excited and terrified at the same time. My body is not what it was; but I'm ready to accept there are things I will genuinely struggle with (being still for one!). It's all part of a learning curve I'm experiencing, a real understanding that I am so different now. Each of us is unique yes, but at any given moment, what you thought was yours permanently can be gone in the blink of an eye. I'm lucky, I'm positive I'll be back to my old self by the end of the year, but with a deeper sense of empathy. I will cherish any pose that my body can handle tonight, and am forever grateful I'm rolling my mat out again; with a bright future still ahead of me.

THE CANCER PATIENT

20th April 2017

The Yoga Sutras

"Yogas Chitta Vritta Nirodha" (Yoga Sutras Chapter 1, verse 2.)

This has been on my mind all week and longer to be totally honest. If you were to Google it, it would probably translate from Sanskrit as "Yoga is to control the modifications of the mind". In my book it says "to block the patterns of consciousness is yoga."

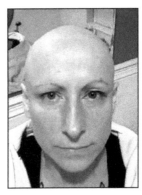

Slowly but surely I am beginning to see the cancer patient emerge before my eyes in the mirror; and I can do nothing to prevent it. I lie in the bath, and there she is looking back at me. I don't know who she is yet, but this poor creature is me. I have laughed and I have cried at this image; an image that I am more used to seeing on the television in adverts and films. The reality that this is me is overwhelming and all consuming. This has brought me close to the edge of that proverbial 'cliff' many times in the last 8 days, but on each occasion, this simple Sanskrit statement (and the incredible people around me) has kept me from getting any closer. I have realised, more than ever, I must be able to control the changes going on in my mind. Changes trying to pull me back into a place I know all too well.

As I have mentioned, 7 years ago I suffered from severe depression and became suicidal. I was under the care of counsellors, doctors, nurses, psychologists, all trying to help me

22

piece a shattered self-back together again. I jumped headfirst off that cliff...I know it, every inch of it in fact. It is only by the grace of God (or fate, or whatever) that am I here today. I say it all the time... I am one of the luckiest people in the world, and I really do mean it! I actually threw my life away, but I was handed it right back. The universe screamed at me, NO! It is not your time to go! I was forced to face up to my biggest fears, whether I wanted to or not. I had to metaphorically learn to crawl again, stand up, walk, run and fight for an existence I didn't even think I deserved. I fought and I won. (That is a whole other story.) Since then, I've continued winning and passing on those skills to others for years. So what the hell in the last week went so wrong? What pushed me to the edge again?

Simple, I underestimated all of this: the C word, the chemo, the steroids, the needles, the sickness, the pain, the darkness, the fears, the desperation, the part of it all that makes you think you're dying. The whole irony of it all, because this time, I didn't want to! This time I wanted to live! How bloody unfair was that? Was someone taking the piss? I'd laughed in the face of cancer, snarled at it, "I've been in worse places, don't underestimate me, you don't frighten me." And cancer smacked me right back in the face saying, "Don't underestimate me either!"

OK, so now I know. I'm ill, I'm in a scary place I know nothing about, with no reference points from my own past to guide me. I accept that some days will be as bad as places I've been before, I get it. Sometimes (as you'll see by the picture) I have no control over things that may happen to my face or my body. I am human. I am vulnerable. But my mind, that's mine. I can control that. I have so much to learn, still. I am learning to control my mind; and this was what yoga was always about for me. It was never the headstands, the fitness, the diets, even the teaching: but a place in my own head of contentment and peace. As they say in yoga, 'Santosha'.

My biggest lesson that returned to face me this week, I have no right ever to doubt my own worth, my own existence, (or that of anyone else's either.) None of us have. I shouldn't live a life where I think it's my duty to only give to others; I should live and love my life for me. 'Coz I'm worth it'. So cancer.... I win again and you, you little shit, regardless of anything or any outcome- you lose.

27th April 2017

Julie's home from the hospital safe and sound and 'Donald Lump' has gone. (Love her sense of humour!) Her chemo wasn't working, so they stopped it to give her a mastectomy instead of the planned lumpectomy. Once she's gotten over her surgery, she'll be back on chemo again. It's so unfair for her though, her hair is growing back a beautiful white colour and it means she'll lose it again. TN is an absolute bastard, it's meant to be chemo sensitive but that clearly isn't always the case.

28th April 2017

Yesterday a memory came up on my computer, one I remember only too well. I had gone to the doctors and he had spent a good 20 minutes with me. My problem was I had a lump. I had also lost weight dramatically (over a stone) and generally felt something was very wrong. No, he didn't think the lump was anything (bad call), but he did send me for a ton of blood tests. That shocked me to be honest. He also insisted I returned if my lump changed at all. The blood results came back and showed nothing of course. Throughout the year, the lump never changed but everything else fell apart. I had severe bone pain, hip pain, stomach problems, severe back pain, night sweats, and exhaustion. So more blood tests were taken, but they only showed anaemia, and nothing else. I knew though, something was very, very wrong. Then more blood tests, but nothing.

Eventually the lump began to change in November and I went back. I remember visiting a friend a few days after my appointment and having a missed call off the Doctor. When I saw it, my heart sank. I just knew this was the beginning of something really bad. After an ultrasound and biopsy which took place over a month (due to Christmas and New Year slowing appointments down), I was finally given my diagnosis: Triple Negative breast cancer. I was relieved to a degree that it was cancer; it showed my instincts were dead right. All year I had known I was ill, and I was. Cancer was what I feared and cancer was what it was.

So please, please, don't muck about with your body. Listen to it, blood tests don't always show things, and neither do scans. Get to know your body, understand it, and push your doctor if you think something is wrong. It might well save your life. I was so bloody lucky, that lump should have done more damage, but it didn't. (So far as I know anyway.) There but for the grace of God go I, again.

29th April 2017

I'm feeling my new hair growing on top of my head, but still losing it at the back though. I'll keep shaving it until it's ready to grow all over. Eye lashes and eyebrows are thinning too now. They'll be next to go I guess. But do you know what, I don't mind. I'm alive and feel more alive than I ever have done before. The world may want to drag me down, and sometimes it almost does. But I'll keep fighting, smiling and laughing regardless. In the two paths of life, love versus hate, I'll choose love every time. That's why I know, I'll always win.

30th April 2017

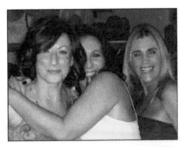

I went out last night with my friends Lynn and Sharon Floweth Brown and I had the absolute best night ever! I have been winding up Lynn for months, saying that once I had a wig on in public, I would muck about with it... and I did. I kept moving it about, trying to get it straight, so it was pretty obvious I was wearing a wig. Lynn dived on me and helped put it straight, then kissed me on the forehead. I danced the night away (with what energy I had), with lipstick on my head. Thanks for that my mad friend, I didn't look ridiculous at all!

2nd May 2017

I had a bit of a heads up today. I woke up this morning and had a bit of pain in my groin, but didn't really think much of it. By lunch, I kept on needing a wee. Then within a few hours I was in agony, burning like hell, feeling like I'd been kicked between the legs and doubled up in pain. So I phoned the hotline and they told me to get the doctors immediately. Result is, I have a bad bladder infection and I'm on antibiotics but I can't believe the speed at which it took hold. I've no idea if they will still fit my Hickman line tomorrow or if I will be able to have my first Taxol on Thursday. I can only hope. Clearly I am more vulnerable than I thought.

3rd May 2017

Today I had my Hickman Line fitted. This will mean I will no longer need to have a cannula inserted or bloods removed with a needle each time I am having chemo. Lynn came with me to my last oncologist appointment, and we all discussed which line would be best for me. It has been awful having a cannula every time for the EC, I was in so much pain with it. I knew there was no way I could cope with a cannula for Taxol 9 times and blood being taken weekly too!

So today, it's gone in. It is the most invasive type of line, but the most effective. I'll be honest, it was absolutely awful! I'm in a lot of pain from the cuts in my neck and chest and spent the whole journey home crying, thinking what the hell have I done to myself now? At home I couldn't even move my head, lie down or even sleep. I feel like someone has cut my neck and chest to pieces. I'm telling myself over and again, it's only temporary and better than the alternative! It won't be forever, I know.

4th May 2017

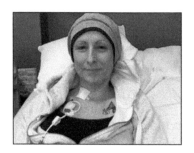

So here I am with my line. I'm onto Paclitaxol now (also known as Taxol). The first one has gone in, and I have 8 left weekly over the next 2 months. After the hell of yesterday, I can't believe how much easier this line is! I was in agony yes, but it was so worth it today. I simply lay there on one of the beds, (I've been looking forward to that), got hooked up... and went to sleep. I don't care that it's restrictive, uncomfortable and still hurts, it's so much easier. I feel crap but genuinely so happy. I win again.

7th May 2017

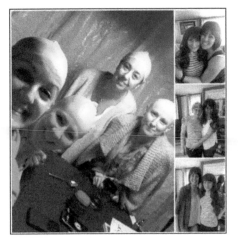

I have just had the best few days with some friends of mine who used to be neighbours, Juliette Blower, Rachael Judd and Wendy Pike. I think between us we have seen a lot of life! We stayed at my friend Juliette's caravan in the Lake District. It was so wonderful just to get away; and try at least to be normal. I must admit, the Hickman Line was worrying me a lot though, and I couldn't leave it alone. Eventually, Rachael told me off for messing with it! We had loads of fun trying on my different wigs (I think I have a problem because I have far too many now). It's fab how a wig can change your face so easily. In the evening, they all disappeared for a bit to give me a surprise... I had no idea what was coming. Then they all trouped in wearing skull caps: it was hilarious! We sat there all night, me bald and them wearing their caps; it was such a lovely way of making me feel comfortable. Thanks girls.

8th May 2017

To Give and To Receive

This morning I decided to do my cards (they are called the Goddess Guidance Oracle Cards by Doreen Virtue Ph.D.). I've found they often speak to me. And again they did.

As most people know, I absolutely love my job teaching yoga. The hours I've spent teaching have brought so much pleasure to me, but it's not just that. I love seeing the change in people, seeing them realise if they want, they can make changes in their life. I do it because I want to help; it's my 'dharma' (duty). I want people to see there is more to them than they can ever imagine. In my own little world, I want to make a difference and see the ripples flow. I want to spread love, acceptance, kindness, the list goes on! Yet, when it comes to me, I often find it hard to receive it back. Maybe it's guilt, I don't know? Maybe that feeling of- 'but I'm meant to be helping you?' Then today I pull out this card, Hathor, and I am told straight- it's all about balance. (You call upon Hathor, an Egyptian Goddess, to nurture and guide. She is a motherly figure.) They are telling me I need to fill myself up again; I must receive before I am able to give.

As I began writing this morning, it was about insurance of all things, critical illness and life insurance cover. I had it once and foolishly got rid of it because I figured I was tempting fate... only 6 months before all this. (Bad call!) Suddenly realising you have nothing; completely relying on family, friends and the kindness of strangers is very humbling. I am learning to receive with grace, humility and so much gratitude. I have been the recipient of overwhelming kindness and generosity. (My heartfelt thanks goes to the abundance of people, family, friends, yogis and yoginis out there, who have laid petals at my feet and made this path easier to tread). Unfortunately, we live in a world where money is needed, (so I do l intend to win the lottery!) Until then, I rely on the state and kindness and I know I am blessed.

What I would urge you to do: if you don't have cover or if you aren't entitled to a decent sickness pay- then do something about it and do it now. Please, it would be one less thing for you to worry about if anything ever happened. It is not tempting fate as I once thought... it is simply using your common sense. Worrying about money during a traumatic time in your life; is the last thing you need!

11th May 2017

Woo hoo, it's very sparing, but my hair is growing back! Not shaving it because of a bang to my head did me a favour; I can see what's happening now. I'm going to stick to the clippers while still on this chemotherapy, and until it's thicker. Then I'll let it grow. (Hee, hee, it's the small things.) It is so wonderful to have a cool head though, and ditch the wigs for a bit. Wigs are fab, but they are hot. There are lots of little things I have left from surgery too: 'a blue tit' (I am still a Smurf); numbness from where they removed lymph nodes, and I only seem to sweat on one armpit! In this recent heat, I feel like I'm half soaked, very bizarre…

15th May 2017

I've just had a wonderful morning and afternoon at Wyvale Garden Centre in Bolton again with Julie and Cath. (We are the Three Amigos!). We had a fabulous time putting the world to rights, (they should put us three in charge of this country I think.) Then to add to such a fab time, the waitress came over with free drinks for us; because we'd been talking for so long. I don't think we came up for air to be honest! There was so much we had to discuss and we never stopped. They must have known we were all on treatment, so they gave us a little treat. How fantastic is that? Free brews because we talk so much! We definitely need to come here more often.

18th May 2017

Sleep Is My Best Friend

I slept through my chemo today, the ease of my line gave me that option and I am so glad I made that call to have it fitted. I'm on the chemotherapy drug Paclitaxol now, which I'm given weekly over 9 weeks (6 to go) and I have been blown away to find out that it originates from the beautiful Yew tree. *(Hence the second chapter in this book being called The Red Death and The Yew Tree...I bet you wondered about that one.)*

Thousands of years ago, the Yew Tree was used by the Romans for snake bites. Going back further in India (Ayurvedic medicine); the Yew Tree was used to treat stomach cancers. Now here I am, in 2017, being treated for cancer, with a chemotherapy that has been developed from knowledge gained thousands of years ago. It would seem that we have a lot to learn from the past and Eastern medicine.... It makes me ache, yes, makes me very tired, yes, but so far, I'm coping well. There's a reason for this: I rest, I sleep, I pace myself and most importantly, I'm not working. I do get out for a few hours at a time, and everyone sees me at my very best. Then I go home.... and I sleep. Often I sleep for a whole day. Even a visit from a friend will send me after to my bed; sleep has become my best friend!

I found the last drug EC, however, debilitating. It made me at times prefer death to the treatment itself. If I ever need it in the future, I will say no. Not a chance. Even though I knew it was temporary; I also knew that was it, never ever again. And this is the thing... no matter how hard I look for an answer, I don't know if my cancer will return. I don't know if I will ever need chemo again. Statistically, Triple Negative has a higher risk of metastasis (the cancer spreading). If this happens, you become a 'cancer lifer'. You will need treatment for the rest if your life, and all too often, a shorter one. I have obviously gone over this possibility in my mind over and again... I'm human.

Two days ago I spend hours searching Dr Google for the answer. Will this happen to me? Am I going to die in 5 years or so? Will the chemo not have been able to kill all of the rogue cells? Is it spreading now? How can I find out? How can I find an answer? Then I realised, what a complete and utter bloody waste of 2 hours. I'd have been better off sleeping! But it gave me more than that, I'm an extremely positive person and a huge penny dropped. So what if it returned, it will all be happening perfectly if it did, whatever comes? But that was in the future, not now; and I was looking to a future I can't predict. So I had to pull it back, look to right now, here, this moment in time. I had to control my mind. 'Yoga Chitta Vritta Nirodha'

I stood at the back door and watched the rain fall on the leaves of the sycamore trees, transfixed by the stunning green of the leaves and I laughed at myself. I realised, it was all good, whatever happened. Honestly. Then I made my decision. I would give myself 5 years to live and I would live it well. In 5 years, I would achieve so much. I would return to India next year, study Yoga Therapy and Reiki, and find a way to help people further than I had ever imagined. I've changed my life around in 5 years before; the next 5 will be a breeze. So, I'll believe I have 5 years to live for now; my own words, my own choice. Then of course, when that time is up.... I'll simply give myself another 5. Over and over again I'll do this and I'll live each and every day well. When I'm 90 and I look back, I'll see how lucky I was to have chosen to live that way. So, may my first 5 years continue to be full of these blessings I've received. Thank you cancer, you've been a gift.

24th May 2017

Ariana Grande Bombing

The last few days have been a shock to all of us and completely devastating for far too many. Bombing a concert where children will be attending is beyond comprehension. I cannot even begin to imagine what so many will be going through. Heart-breaking doesn't come even close. Yesterday I found it difficult to read as the different victims were named, like so many of you, my empathy went into overdrive. I thanked God that neither of my girls had been there, as so many of us will have done. All day, the only thing I felt I could do was send my love, thoughts and prayers, to all of those in pain, suffering, in shock. The prayer I chose to use was Metta (Loving Kindness prayer), please do search it and try it. It's a well-known meditation and if every day, every person practised this, I think the world would change. I know we are a long way from that, but I'm an idealist person, and I live in hope.

26th May 2017

The Sun is Out!

Doesn't it make a difference when the sun comes out? Have you noticed what happens? You suddenly become so much more in the moment. This has been a week from hell for so many, (my thoughts and love still go to them all). Then the sun comes and we're all so thankful and grateful for what we have.

Why do we have to wait for that? We seem to spend our lives waiting: waiting for the weekend, for our holidays, for good weather, for Christmas, for our retirement. We get through bad days in the hope that the thing we're waiting for will make it all worth it. Why do we have to wait for the sun, or for something devastating to make us look deeper, be more appreciative of what we already have? And how long will we keep that frame of mind, to remain forever grateful? Will we remember what we have learnt this week; how we've seen strangers come together to help, support, show kindness and love? Will we forget when the sun disappears, or will we remember this lesson. To appreciate every moment we are blessed with, come rain or shine.

I can't go in the sun at the moment, figures eh? This chemo makes me very light sensitive. So I bought a hat weeks ago in anticipation of some sunshine, forever hopeful of the British summer. The tag said £7 but at the till, she charged me £2; I shot out of that shop like a bullet! You would have thought I'd won the Lottery, not saved £5 in a sale. Today I got to sit out in it;

technically I was in the shade, under my new hat. I had a lovely time with my beautiful yoga instructor of old, Callie Meakin and her little dog Chester. Always she will be to me, the woman who showed me the path which ultimately would change my life.

I've been so lucky and blessed by the help and support I'm getting from so many. When I see people, talk to people, it literally brings me sunshine. In that short space of time, I get to be normal again, talk and share normal problems. I know after, it often sends me to bed to recover and rest, but that's ok. I honestly appreciate every word, thought, prayer, text, visit, like it's another sunny day for me. And I remember, I remember how lucky I truly am. I wouldn't change a thing.

27th May 2017

Thank you so much for all your support, again! Every person's kindness and support makes this journey 100 times easier. Katya, Donna, and everyone who continues to lift me and keep me up, I wouldn't be able to do this without you: beautiful souls, thank you.

6th June 2017

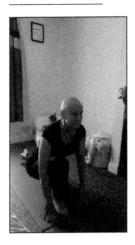

I have been sensible, I have been patient, I have waited and waited. I truly have been so kind, gentle and mindful with my body. At times this has killed me and led me into real bouts of depression. I look at myself and don't recognise the person staring back at me. That crazy yogi girl just felt like she was slipping slowly away. I have never felt so lost in my life as I have done in these last few weeks. Then yesterday a chunk of my eyelashes came out and I was devastated. It was worse than losing my hair. I'd learned to cope with no hair because my eyes had stood out so much... but now they were disappearing too. Even chemotherapy last week brought me to tears, it all felt never ending. The fatigue and pain was becoming soul destroying...

So today I decided it was time: time to fight back, eyelashes or not. My body had had enough of a rest from more difficult poses; I was ready for my first traditional sun salutation and even my first arm balance. My gut told me I was ready... and yes, I only managed a little, but I did it! The warrior is beginning to find her feet again.

9th June 2017

Here I am, wide awake Googling. And not even about cancer! Today I saw my oncologist and thanks to me clearly being ill yesterday with abdominal pain; I was taken seriously. (I had back, pelvis, abdominal pain, bloating, night sweats, you name it last year and bugger all took me seriously, until they found my cancer.)

So today I was sent for an x-ray and my oncologist could see that my digestive system isn't moving much; so she gave me Movicol to help. Cool, I'm happy. Then I'm looking at my x-ray and I notice something odd: 2 small things on my left side and I question it. That must be the metal she says, on your trousers. I said ok and left.

Tonight, I'm thinking about what she said, and go to examine the linen pants I had on... no metal, weird. Then I twig, I was sterilized years ago with clips. Then the penny drops... they were both together high on my left side? What the hell, surely they should be one on each side? So I Google, 'filshie clips' they're called and in 25% of women they fall off, migrate and can cause pain! Oh my god, so now I know I have a metal clip floating around inside me and maybe that's what caused all of my hip/pelvis/back pain. Another trip to the doctors I guess then...

11ᵗʰ June 2017

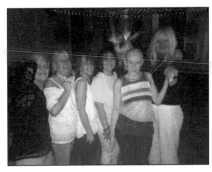

Thank you all so much for last night at the Elvis do. It was an amazing night and I can't thank you Wendy and Ann enough for the whole thing. I loved every second and thanks to all your energy, lasted nearly all night! I had the best time dancing with Lynn to Elvis songs; nothing beats a bit of Elvis. Even my ex-husband came and my girls; it's so wonderful how everyone has come together to support me. My students, family and friends never ever cease to amaze me. I know not everyone could make it, but I am feeling so blessed and your kindness is truly appreciated, you can't imagine.

14ᵗʰ June 2017

It's 5 months after my lumpectomy and sentinel node biopsy and I'm still numb all around my under arm scar, over quite a large area. I seriously thought it would have all gone by now and I am hoping it won't be permanent! I must say, it's so bizarre being able to pinch myself and feel nothing. I must remember to keep away from razors!

16ᵗʰ June 2017

I met up again with Julie for a brew and a good chin wag, as we always do. We were missing our third 'amigo' though because Cath is having her chemo today. We are both going to be on the same chemo now, Paclitaxol. It's not quite as bad as EC was, but it does build up in the system slowly. I've only got a few left thank god; it feels crazy that it's coming to the end! Julie's treatment has all been put back now because the EC wasn't working on her tumour. They've given her a mastectomy instead of a lumpectomy, so today she was fiddling a lot with her fake boob to get it comfortable! (It has a tendency to ride up and it's driving her mental.) This of course also means that she'll lose her hair twice, what a total bastard this disease is. It feels especially unfair, as her hair has grown back such a beautiful silvery white. Everyone seems to have a different protocol when it comes to treatment too; some people have the chemo before surgery and some have it afterwards- we're all so different. I suppose the positive in having the chemotherapy first, is that you know if it works!

I think we must be keeping these local places going with our visits, I might add. It is invaluable when we get together, it truly is.

23rd June 2017

I've had the worst day on Taxol I've ever had. I've cried, I've slept and I've thought 'What is the point?' for most of the day. Then I got a message off my youngest. She was at a wedding with her boyfriend, so she sent me a picture of them both to cheer me up. I would do anything for my two girls. If they said chop off your right arm, that would help, I would. So maybe it's not pointless after all. Thanks Munchkin. (She'll love me for that!)

29th June 2017

Well....here it is, the morning of my last chemo. I'm up and about to put a 'face' on so I look 'normal'. Not that I care to be fair. I have had 4 months of poison in my system, 6 months of 'cancer' in my life and the second stage of treatments is about to end. I have very mixed emotions, but to be honest, I am amazed at a strength I never knew I had.

As the last few drops of my chemo went in this afternoon, 'I can see clearly now' played on the radio. More poignant words I couldn't have chosen myself. I got to ring the bell too of course. There is a poem for you to read out before you ring the bell, and this was considerably harder than I thought it would be! I was in tears by the end of it. God, how emotional was today. I am stunned and amazed that I made it.

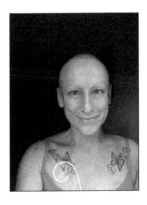

A POET EMERGES

1st July 2017

Fully Charged... Me, Then and Now

So chemo has ended and a new journey is beginning. I've wanted to write so many times in the last few weeks, but have had no energy to do so. I can best describe myself as a phone and a charger. How often have you had to charge your phone in a rush only to get 20%, and then wonder why it runs out so fast? That's me. I have to recharge more often and if I don't give my body a decent length of charge, all I'm going to get is 20% max. Even fully charged, I only get 50%. It's a new body I'm learning to live with and accept. For now it can't do half the things it could do 6 months ago, but hell, I'm alive!

I'm beginning to dip into some classes now, and I'm desperate to say thank you for so much support and to get my strength back! I'm nowhere near ready for teaching though. I haven't even had radiotherapy yet; but I am beginning my road to recovery. I look different, my abilities are different, my body is different... however, my wish to be as daft and disruptive as possible hasn't diminished! I can't kneel down, so kneeling poses are out the window. Down dog is a 'no no' until my line is out too, but I'm patient. I have no choice but to be! I know I will get there in the end.

I've learnt much on this journey, but the thing I have cherished and loved the most is the kindness, love, support and generosity I've received. So many people have been there for me: my mum, my family, my friends, and many of my students. There has also been a wealth of yoga instructors who covered my classes, alongside hundreds of people who went out of their way to support me. You have no idea what it has meant to me, I am forever grateful. You all know who you are! The day will come when I can both thank you all and repay this huge kindness. Of that, I am sure.

The best way I can repay you for now is to heal, build my strength and get back into classes. Prove to you all that this shit disease won't break me; pass on what I'm learning and show you how you can fight and win!

3rd July 2017

I'm having a Marvellous Monday! My line is out, chemo is over and I'm enjoying a meal and a glass of spiced rum. (Captain Morgan's of course, no Fanta Lemon though Lynn!) When the nurse finally took out my line, I literally ran out of the hospital; they were in stitches at my excitement. I nearly took out a few nurses on my way! Oh, the food is totally fab here too. Can't believe I can actually eat that much now, thanks chemo.

10th July 2017

It's Not Over Until I Win

And so chemo has finished, woo hoo! I spent most of last week pretty much excited, thinking thank God for that: I survived! On Monday, I even went into a class to deliver the meditation and was made up to see so many. In the afternoon I had the Hickman line removed and despite it being a longer process than she anticipated; the nurse congratulated me on having strong healing skin and tissue. (How smug was I... Hmmm is that ego a quiet voice whispered to me?) By Tuesday night, I was sure I'd be in a headstand by the end of the following week: after the stitches had dissolved of course and my miraculous skin had healed.

What a week it was becoming, my head was way, way ahead of everything, I genuinely felt nothing could stop me. On Wednesday, I had my radiotherapy meeting. I had researched it well I thought, so was ready to sign my life away- again. I was pleased I'd have a month before it started though. Even in my crazy positive mind (that was now preparing to test the waters with a wealth of advanced poses); I knew my body needed to rest, build strength, recover, and recuperate from chemotherapy. I listened to her explain the side effects:

✓ Sunburn, check- I knew that
✓ More boob shrinkage, check- (crap yeah), but I knew that
✓ Swelling of the breast, check- I knew that
✓ Hair loss in the arm pit, check- woo hoo, I knew that!
✓ Pain in the chest/breast, check- (not good) but I knew that
✓ Tiredness and fatigue, check- used to that anyway
✓ Muscle deterioration in the chest... pardon?
✓ Bone weakness in the ribs...what!?

I'll be honest, I felt like I'd been punched in the chest initially. It actually hit me harder than my initial diagnosis, how strange is that? All of these images of me upside down challenging myself in headstands, handstands, crow... came crashing down in one fell swoop. I looked at her like she had the wrong person, had got it wrong, and was talking absolute rubbish. I composed myself and made my point, "I'm a yoga instructor so I'll be building back up soon to my former fitness levels." I even described the poses I intended to do. She looked at me, like I was the mad one, "You will not get back to your previous fitness levels for about 12 months, after radiotherapy." Oh, right, I thought, so much for the headstand... but it was only going to be a baby one, I swear!

It was funny when I got back in the car, I felt like I'd landed firmly back on my feet, (or my backside to be correct); back to the reality I was in. I'm a cancer patient, albeit a wonder woman warrior type version; but a cancer patient all the same. I thought about what she had said. I realised how lucky I was to be alive to be fair and to know there would still be an end eventually to this crap. I still loved my life when all was said and done.

My week went on. I met my wonderful Warrior friends on Thursday, who are all on the same journey as me. Julie and Cath and I, the 'Three Amigos', putting the world to rights as we so often do. Again, I may have been tired by this point and a little down from pushing myself too much (when will I learn eh?): but, come on, I was alive and ready to fight. My week still wasn't over.... I was back to common sense by Saturday and I rested, all day. Then Sunday arrived, and I spent it with some of my students, overwhelmed again by their kindness and love. There is no lesson I have learnt more throughout this, than the pure, love, empathy and beauty in people. I could repay everyone with the world, and it still wouldn't be enough.

And so I begin another week. My chemo has ended, yes, but I began another journey last night. I began the journey of the after effects of chemo; what we call 'SE', the side effects. Of course, I've had many already: but don't be fooled into thinking after chemo- that's it, it's done. It's not, not by a long shot. I've begun with peripheral neuropathy in my hands and feet and last night was a living hell. My feet and hands are constantly tingling, twitching, in pain and some-times numb. The Paclitaxol has destroyed my nervous system, and I pray to God I'm on the temporary side of statistics. I truly hope that it fades over the next few months... or there may have to be many more changes in my life. But, despite anything still yet to come, it's not over till I win. Just watch me; I will be back in those baby headstands before you know it!

13th July 2017

The Voices

I currently have different voices in my head... that of Edwina the yoga instructor, that of Edwina the cancer patient and then, just Edwina the mad one who takes whatever life throws at her and plays with it.

The mad one is saying, 'I'm bored playing this game now, had enough with the whole cancer and chemotherapy malarkey. I want to go back to normal... like right now! '

The yoga instructor is saying, 'Go gently girl, listen to that body, let go of that ego, respect what has happened to your body, to your 'vehicle' and practise what you have been preaching for the last 6 years. Do you ever actually learn?'

Then there's the cancer patient, she's the worst of them all. She's stamping her feet saying, 'What the f**k has happened to this body? I didn't sign up for this? I'm doing a handstand right now... try and bloody stop me!'

I literally am a wealth of feelings, emotions, thoughts and ideas. On one hand I'm determined; on the other I'm cautious. I'm brazen and terrified both at the same time. I'm different, I'm learning all over again. I'm desperate to return to what I do best, but I have to get my strength first. I am no longer the yoga instructor with an impressive control of her body; I'm simply that kid in the corner doing her own thing.

15th July 2017

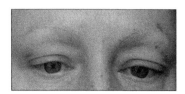

The joys of chemotherapy: finding out in the morning that more eyebrow lashes fell out when you cleaned your face last night. Only on the one side of course, where's the fun in being even! Eyebrow pencil, where are you? Not even sure where start without a guide.

20th July 2017

The Never Ending Journey

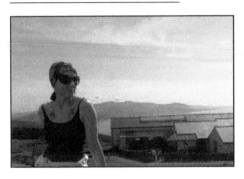

I've just returned from the best 3 days I've had in months. 3 days in Llandudno and I actually feel like I've been away for a week. It couldn't have been better. The weather was perfect, the hotel and room were amazing, and the views were stunning. For those 3 days I got to escape! I was so blessed, walks on the prom and Pier, two trips up and around the Great Orme, a visit to my old school town of Rhos-on-Sea; and yesterday a trip to Conway. I think my step counter is in shock, it probably didn't know I was capable!

It's funny when you go away, because you know you have to come back to reality. It's never good is it? In your head you're thinking, I've got to go back to work and I really don't want to! It's different for me. Yes I'm thinking I've got to prepare again for returning in the future, but I'm thinking more of the next course of treatment: the radiotherapy to come. I'll admit, I'm now very apprehensive about it. Having spent so long in the sun (with Factor 50 cream on I add), I've still had a severe allergic reaction to it. My skin is so sensitive from chemo, it's on fire. God alone knows how radiotherapy will affect it. But I've got to push that aside and focus on nearer things to come.

Everything has helped me to make another decision, something I've wanted to do in so long... I'm getting a puppy, a whippet. He comes in a few weeks and will no doubt drive me mad! He will keep my mind occupied, be a distraction from it all, and give me unconditional love as animals do. More importantly he'll help me recover quicker and be a part of my family for a long, long time. It's not a decision I've made lightly and it's all go now to prepare for him! The decisions we make in times of crisis are often our best I think. During my time off work years ago, in one of my darkest moments I booked a trip to India to train as a yoga instructor. I had no doubt it was right, I followed my instincts and it worked out so well. So maybe people think I'm mad with this one, but trust me.

One thing I have also needed to do for months is write a poem. Yes, a poem, not something I ever saw coming I'll be honest! I think I've always had the writer's 'app', just never actually used it much. I've needed to let go of how this all feels for months and escaping gave me that chance to really let it go. You see, just because chemo ends, doesn't mean it's over. I still have the side effects; I still have to deal with them, every day. And sometimes it's harder than others. Yet these words are not just about me, they belong to so many others out there.

Anyone who knows this journey will tell you, it feels never ending. Every day during chemotherapy treatment and since, I wake up and immediately see my face. (Unfortunately, mirrored wardrobes mean that I can't escape my image.) When my eyelashes and eyebrows fell out, that was as much as I could take. For those who are there, I know how you feel. For me, I still have radiotherapy to come and 5 years of wondering if my cancer is still growing in my body somewhere, yet I'm one of the lucky ones. So I leave you with my words on how this all feels... Who Am I?

<u>Who Am I?</u>

I look in the mirror,
But what do I see?
The ghost of the person,
I once thought was me.

My sunken eyes empty.
No lashes or hair.
My brows slowly fading.
In silence, I stare.

So, I search for what's left,
I draw on a face.
I cover my baldness,
All done without haste.

"I'm ready", my voice tells,
This image I've made.
"I know that you're in there,
I won't let you fade..."

"But it grows back!", they say,
Cheap words in the air.
Well, you try it then,
Now that makes it fair...

Don't question my fears and,
Don't tell me to wait!
You have to live through this,
To know of my fate.

I try to be happy,
I laugh and I smile.
All through this false image,
I hold for a while.

But inside, I'm broken,
A battle each day;
To carry this disguise,
And not hide away.

So next time you see me,
With 'wisdom' to share...
Remember I'm struggling,
With just being there.

I've looked in the mirror,
This morning and seen,
A shell of the person,
That I had once been.

Edwina Maria Thompson
© 2017

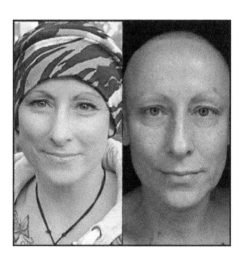

21st July 2017

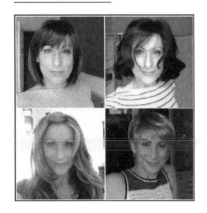

She's at it again! I've only gone and bought myself ANOTHER wig… I have about 5 of them now. I have to admit, buying wigs has been a little bit like therapy for me, and I have loved wearing every single one of them. 'Simply Wigs' even have me on their website. They really do make me feel more 'normal', and I can be a different person every time. This latest one is a short blonde, and it looks fab! No one would ever know.

I had the best night out with Lynn in this latest wig a few days back. We danced late into the night, but when I got too hot- I just took it off! I carried on dancing, with a bald head, wig in hand and I genuinely didn't care. Then suddenly loads of people came up to give me a hug. One lady was in tears to see me, as her sister had just died of cancer. Simply to watch me well and enjoying myself, gave her hope that life can go on after cancer. Yet again, I am overwhelmed at the kindness of strangers. It still touches me now just to think of the power in the hug she gave me. Someone I had never met.

Regards my wigs though, this has got to be the last one. Enough is enough; you'd think I had a problem! How cool are they all though?

24th July 2017

Life Is So Very, Very Short.

We often forget how fragile our lives are because we get so wrapped up in the world around us. We run around like idiots, following the rules, doing as we're told, being the person everyone expects us to be. I've been there myself and that world eventually broke me and nearly killed me. I know I will never go back there again, thank God! I escaped. I had the opportunity to change my life due to the dire circumstances around me, but it actually turned out to be a blessing in disguise. It couldn't have turned out more perfectly.

I was once asked by a doctor- who did I think I was? My answer... 'I'm a mother, a wife, a teacher, a friend, a daughter, a sister'... the list went on. He looked at me and said, 'No, who are you? What do you want in life, what do you do for you?' I was stunned, I cried, I couldn't answer him. I had no idea. In moulding myself to every role I was playing, I had lost all identity of myself. I didn't have a clue who I was anymore and as a result of that loss of myself, I plunged further into depression. It took yoga to pull me back out. But that doesn't mean yoga is my life, far from it. It is simply the crutch and support by which I live my life. It helped me to find out who I was. It gave me strength, confidence and self-worth again.

Today I went to visit Neo. I only have to look at him and he melts my heart in every way. The joy I feel is so real, it radiates from me. I have wanted a dog for years, in reality about 20 years; but I couldn't. I was too busy in all my other roles to devote time to a puppy. Yet here I am, coming out of a hellish journey where I couldn't be happier. I'm not daft, I know he will be therapeutic for me, but he will be so, so much more. Yet again, beauty unfolds from the darkness in my live.

I have had cancer and it's shit, really shit. Finding out is only the start. Surgery, treatments and recovery are not a 'walk in the park'. Too frequently I'm learning of beautiful strong women with my type of cancer who have passed away. I don't want to be negative about it, but it's the truth- the real, awful, cruel and brutal truth. In reality, in every hundred women with my cancer, probably about 20 and possibly more will die within 5 years or so. (To be honest, statistically it's more than that, but I'm being positive here as more research is being made.) They leave behind babies, children, husbands, family, friends and it's devastating. It is not a pink heart or a post on a wall- it's pain, tears, heartbreak and loss. Nothing less.

I see so many of us still falling into the trap of thinking we have forever. Well, we don't, do we? Why do we think we have? Who has ever told us that we're going to live forever? I am alive and incredibly grateful for that. I have the biggest smile on my face thanks to those who gave love to someone in a bad place. I know I am blessed now; cancer pulled me up and reminded me that my time on earth is precious. So now, I'm asking everyone to remember 'you' too. What are you missing out on? What do you really want in life? Life is short and we aren't here forever. Don't wait for something like cancer or any other hell to give you the push... if you have a Bucket or a Life List, get on it! You have this life right now, so please god don't waste it away. It is no one else's responsibility to make you happy, or make any changes- it's yours. So find that smile of pure light and love and send it to yourself.

25th July 2017

After an amazing day yesterday, I fell back into reality last night at yoga. I might add, the excitement over Neo will continue to put a smile on my face though! Basically, I really struggled with some of my favourite poses, warrior and tree. It's due to the peripheral neuropathy in my hands and feet, but particularly my hands. It means my hands tingle most of the time and in poses where I raise my hands, they become numb. (It's like when you've lain on your arm too long and you can't feel any sensation properly). Hopefully it will wear off; it's early days and I haven't even started my next treatment yet.

My body is different, I am different, and my abilities are different. My teaching therefore is going be different. Honestly, I'm terrified. I'm probably not ready physically, mentally or emotionally to teach yet and I've no idea as yet how it will feel. In warrior last night, I could have cried because my hands were so uncomfortable. My balance is affected too... I feel like I'm on a paddle board doing water yoga! I literally have zero balance skills right now.

Maybe I'm not as fit as I was, damaged in places still; a little like my 'new' car Phoenix. But like her, if I go gently: there are still many miles left on the clock.

26th July 2017

And so, from a diagnosis on January 6th 2017, investigations that began in April of 2016, I have been handed the date of my final 'active' treatment. This is the date that marks the beginning of the end... August 23rd 2017. I wonder what I'll be doing this time next year?!

28th July 2017

What a fabulous Friday we have just had. Today I met up with some warriors, Julie of course, Debbie Roocroft and Shirley Mather. We had a lovely afternoon as always. I do love our 'get togethers', they make you feel 'normal!' Julie has a new wig and looks fabulous (as always!). It's a soft grey colour and looks completely natural; you just would never know. It only cost her £10 on eBay too. I think I need to get on there now; mine all cost an arm and a leg!

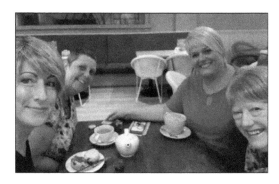

6th August 2017

Gratitude

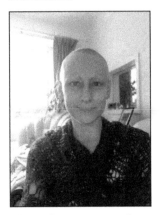

I've had a fab few days catching up with friends and family this weekend, (regardless of being tired.) An old friend Vicky Gorst-Smith said something to me on Friday that really touched me and fired me up. Then today I saw my wonderful cousins David Thompson and Catherine Thompson, my Aunty Angela and Uncle Mike, (and my brother and Mum too). I've been so blessed to receive love and kindness in so many ways over the last months. Then David presented me with a beautiful gift of a purple crochet shawl he had made for me in a peacock pattern to protect me! How perfect is that.

On Friday, Vicky said how she had prepared herself to see 'Edwina with cancer', not having seen me in a year. As she explained, seeing photos is different to actually seeing a person face to face. But seeing me, talking to me, I was still me, Edwina. The cancer simply faded in comparison to me. I was bigger than the cancer. For those of you still there, never forget that!

That's it isn't it? That regardless of everything we ever encounter, we are always more than we can ever imagine. Our spirit, soul, essence, (whatever you want to call it), is invincible! Life may throw an immense amount of crap our way, devastating at times: we may at times wonder, why me? Why did this happen to me? This wasn't my path! This is unfair! But that is life isn't it... there is good and there is bad. It's what we take from it that makes us. Like my cousin Catherine said, it's the positives we take.

This has brought my thoughts to a film I saw years ago, 'The Matrix' with Keano Reeves. (Yes that is where Neo's name came from, Keano's character.) In the film, people were linked to a computer programme which gave them the appearance of a real world. In reality, they were being used as human batteries. The world that was created for them was perfect... no illness, no death, no crime, no hate; but it didn't work. It crashed, simply because the people didn't believe in it: perfect wasn't a reality!

We need the darkness, difficulties, and pain; only then do we truly appreciate the light. It's in our darkest times that we really learn, grow and evolve. I am more blessed than I ever imagined, I am surrounded by love from every angle. It surrounds me and protects me. It is my constant reminder that "I am bigger than this." I know that I am truly grateful for every experience I have; and when I am grateful... it naturally keeps me content. Santosha as always.

12th August 2017

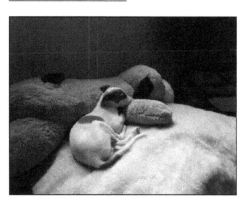

Well, here he is. Meet Neo. He is like Velcro at the moment! So far he has managed to miss every mat put down bar one. I didn't have to mop up this much wee when the girls were little! He loves the big toy dog on his mattress too, and has fallen asleep on it a few times. He truly is adorable! He's just gone to wake up and realised it was all just too much effort. I can't believe how utterly blessed I am to have him. Even my calendar knew it was a special day today.

15th August 2017

Nearly There

7 days left and I am very much aware that the end of the roll-ercoaster is nearly here. A friend of mine from my teaching days, Trish Grogan, has been giving me a lift to hospital daily recently. (I can't tell you how wonderful that is to have support as it's daily trips for 3 weeks, I am so grateful!) I've been chatting to her about the whole 'cancer' thing. Explaining how I was simply coming to another part of my cancer journey, the end of treatment: what is often the hardest part. Most of us think, (as I did before cancer turned up,) that you are given a scan at the end of treatment that will indicate if you are completely free of cancer. This is not the case. There are few oncologists who will say you are fully 'cured', some use NED which is 'no evidence of disease' and 'all clear', but they don't really know 100%.

You would think, wouldn't you, that by the end you would be ecstatic to be there. The truth is, it's a little like jumping off the high jump blindfolded: in the vain hope there's enough water in the pool to keep you safe. I've decided in my own way how to tackle this, as I mentioned early on. I will always live as if I have 5 years (adding on another 5 as I come to the end of the previous 5). It's my way of making sure I make the most of every moment, that I cherish everything I have, have no regrets and enjoy my life! So far, I don't regret a single decision I have ever made. I do appreciate everything I have ever been through, the good, the bad and the hell: because it all brought me here, to right now.

I don't know what is around the corner. I know of too many who had short lives, many of those I knew and loved. I have experienced much in my life already, but if I was destined to die tomorrow of a freak accident or something; I would still feel bloody lucky to have nearly 50 years on my clock! Now that is amazing!

So I finally face my last sessions of cancer treatment. I understand some side effects are yet to come, and that's ok. I plan not to worry too much, (running around after a puppy that wees everywhere is keeping my mind busy!) My biggest aim right now is to get a full night's sleep, but for that, I must be patient. Neo has just become more important than my wishes or worries. Good plan eh, distraction and unconditional love all rolled into one. I refuse to let cancer take any more of my life away. It can do one. I am bigger than it.

21st August 2017

God give me strength! This whole radiotherapy thing is wearing me out. I've spent 6 years of my life slowing my breathing down. Not just shallow breathing into my chest, but utilising all of my lungs. Now I find out, it makes being still for the machine more difficult! Argh! Every day I hear the words… 'Please breathe normally Edwina; try to keep as still as possible.' I feel like I'm hyperventilating lying there, trying to 'breathe normally'! Thank god I only have 2 left…

23rd August 2017

Just another day for most, the end of 7 months of treatment for me, a journey that began only the week after New Year, January 6th. I can hardly even believe it is here, nothing feels real… my feelings are numb to be honest. I'm not happy, sad, elated or relieved, there's nothing. The only thing I can think about doing now is sleeping for a long, long, long time. If I can just get through today without being told I'm not breathing right, I'll be happy I guess. Thank god it's nearly over. I wonder if it will all be as difficult as they say.

30th August 2017

I've just introduced Julie to Neo, and Julie has introduced me to The Pet Place in Bents Garden Centre. I had no idea it even existed; so like I fool I was wandering around looking for Julie, when she was already sat inside. It was great in there though. I could sit there, with Neo on my knee and have a brew. She's not going to bring Biddy until our next meeting though (Julie's dog), as we're not sure if they'll get on! Afterwards, we had a look around at the pet shop. It's a fantastic place to go so I think we'll be back. She was very impressed that my radio-therapy burns are healing already! So far, the beginning of the end has been a breeze.

TREATMENT OVER AND DONE

4th September 2017

Well, Breast Cancer Awareness Month isn't even here yet, and the Pink Hearts have already started. This time last year, when I was asked to share a heart or post some crap about where you keep your handbag... I did so, without a thought to be honest. Little did I know cancer was already growing inside me and that heart or post didn't make me any the wiser. For a moment I felt sympathy for those who have died from breast cancer, but that was it. I didn't immediately run upstairs and check! That's the thing isn't it: we have become so immune to these things that they mean very little unless we have lost someone close to us, or experienced it ourselves. So what is the point in that? How is that heart or post actually going to save more lives? The reality is, it probably won't to the unaffected. I'm sorry if I'm offending anyone, but it's the truth.

If you are ever asked to post a heart to raise awareness for Breast Cancer, go ahead; but please, post something alongside it which will show ladies (and men) what to actually look for. Knowledge is power, and believe me that will raise awareness a lot more effectively!

So.... here we go: my little answer to those hearts. This poem was inspired by the wonderful leader of our Triple Negative Warrior UK group- Carole-Anne Spicer. I read a post she had written about the 'hearts on a wall' and it spurred me to get writing myself. Let's do something that will actually help, and not waste time on pretty hearts and games. In memory of all of those who lost their battle and in the hope for those I can help to save.

(Thank you to Breast Cancer Care for allowing me to use their image.)

A Heart on a Wall

A Heart on a Wall, achieves nothing at all.
It may make you think, but that's gone in a blink.

I get you feel sad, so much loss makes us mad.
And that heart is your way, to remember today.

But please stop right there. Do some more. Don't just share!
Coz that heart on your wall, teaches nothing at all.

It can't show the fear, for each one of us here;
That live in this hell, like a dark, endless well.

It's not a cute game, we will never feel shame.
We all fight from the start, never hide with a heart.

It's scars, tears and pain, losing hair, tubes, disdain,
With burns, sickness and sores. Need I add anymore?

So please when you share, make the people aware.
Make them check, make them know, any knowledge to show.

Be the one who will teach, for those souls you would reach.
Break that chain and be brave, all those people to save.

Search Breast Cancer Care, find this image and share!

And ditch hearts on a wall, make awareness your call.

Edwina Maria Thompson
© 2017

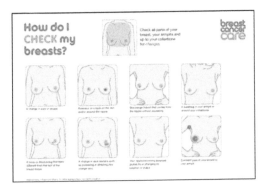

10th September 2017

Aftermath

So it's all come to an end, the rollercoaster of cancer treatment: surgery on January 23rd; a month to recover; 4 months of chemo from March 1st; a month again to recover; radiotherapy during August, ending 7 months to the day of my surgery.

I remember the day of my diagnosis, Jan 6th, less than a week from New Years. I wasn't shocked to be told it was cancer, I was relieved. I just thought, thank god for that, I know what's wrong with me! Now you can bloody well fix me after all this arsing around! In my follow up meeting, I sat and listened to the Breast Cancer nurse explain my type of breast cancer. I looked at her thinking, what the f**k, you mean there are different types? Why don't we all already know this? I'd told everyone, I'll be back in 2 weeks; all they have to do is cut it out... hmmm.

My nurse explained to me what Triple Negative meant, led me through my offered 'standard' treatments: surgery, chemotherapy, radiotherapy. It was just the beginning of a whirlwind, a tornado that was about to suck me in for 7 months, spewing me out at the end: hopefully free of all cancer. I asked the obvious of course, will I lose my hair? Yes was my answer, along with this sympathetic tilt of her head to one side that she must have to do 10 times a day. I remember thinking, but that means I won't finish until August, seriously? We're in January; you are having a bloody laugh! I'll be doing this for the whole of spring and summer? It felt like an alternative reality that I was suddenly in, a parallel universe that had somehow evolved around me. I decided to face it head on, accept everything that was thrown at me, embrace and learn from every lesson I was about to experience. And I have, so far.

I knew from the beginning this was going to be no 'walk in the park'. I knew I would be in pain, lose my hair, eyebrows and eyelashes; have side effects that may well become permanent. I signed my life away 3 times, surgery, chemotherapy, radio-therapy. I laughed at the irony of the chemo side effects, particularly the order in which they were written: 'nausea, death'... There didn't seem much point reading the rest of the side effects as I'd be dead anyway! I faced it all and am here now; spat out of the other side, in remission, NED, (no evidence of disease) with a folder to take away that says 'Moving Forward'.

They warn you afterwards about how you may feel, and you think after all that shit, you'll be ready. I thought I was. Hell, I've survived depression; the aftermath of cancer can't be that hard, can it? If nothing else, I've chosen to be honest with you all. I struggle every single day. Physically I am broken, my body is in a lot of pain from neuropathy and fatigue has hit me hard. Mentally, I'm lost. I feel like I'm waking up every day going, what just happened? (Thank god I have Neo and my incredible family and friends to keep my sanity.) Emotionally, I am exhausted. There are times, like today, I have just cried on and off for no apparent reason other than, I'm tired of it all. Then I have to remember, how lucky I am... I am alive.

A while ago, I was saddened to hear of a young mum with cancer who had been told months after treatment had ended; that her cancer had spread. She was positive but scared and ready to fight. The day came she had to tell her children. I remember feeling devastated for her. How the hell is that right? Can you imagine sitting down and telling your children your time with them is limited? Can you imagine being the one to break your own children's hearts? Can you imagine knowing at the worst time of their life, you aren't there? Can you imagine knowing that you (through absolutely no fault of yours), caused their pain. It was beyond my comprehension! Yet parents are doing exactly that all over the world, every day. I was so mad, that day I wanted to scream at everyone complaining on social media about stupid things. Tell them they didn't know they were effing born!

This whole thing strips you bare, mentally, physically and especially emotionally. You become less patient with selfish behaviour, you want everyone to appreciate how bloody lucky they are. I know I do. There have been too many women who have had to face this hell, and there will continue to be many more. My prayers and love go out to them every day, whoever they may be.

So what have I learnt so far? So many lessons. I know I am far from ready to teach properly. I know I have to look after me first, give my body, mind and heart time to heal. But my main lesson for now is that "Life is a gift". It is so, so precious and it is absolutely not to be wasted. I've spent most of today crying. Maybe I'm grieving for all the mothers, fathers and guardians out there, who have to break their children's hearts. Maybe I'm crying for the loss of me, the person I was. Am I crying for the girl with the long hair who stood on her head and danced like a loon? The girl who now needs help up off the floor from the arthritis in her knees? I don't know. But I do know that while I slowly recover-regain my strength, find my feet again and get some normality back- that from the aftermath a warrior will emerge. A new me, stronger, wiser, tougher, kinder.... and she will never ever forget how bloody lucky she is to be alive, however long that life is to be.

14th September 2017

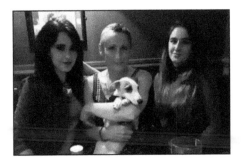

Woo, hoo, it's my birthday! 48 today! I have just had the most wonderful evening out with my partner, two daughters and my youngest's boyfriend. We went to a place where dogs could go, so I could take Neo. He was as good as gold, and only weed once on the floor... (Not sure why I bought a puppy mat to be honest.) Every year, hope against hope, I wonder if my girls will relent and have a picture taken of us all. This year, they couldn't really refuse! (Thank you for that one cancer...) At long last, I have a beautiful picture of the three of us. Might have bloody known they'd wait for me to be practically bald, but I still love it!

2nd October 2017

As I struggle more and more with the side effects of chemotherapy and radiotherapy, it's been forming little rhymes in my mind... and another poem emerged! They are deadly serious when they say that chemotherapy takes you to the very edge and then pulls you back. Everyone is different though, some people suffer badly, and some don't. You can't call it at all-you can only hope. What I do know, is that at times chemo makes you feel like you are dying and that it takes years for the poison to leave your system. I may joke about the side effects, but they genuinely are as bad as they say. Try typing into Google 'chemotherapy se' and watch as a whole list of side effects will pop up. Here are just a few...

The S.E. of C

So now you know what's coming,
Chemotherapy and Rads.
You know that there'll be Side Effects,
You hope they're not too bad!

You sign your life away next,
Not an easy choice to make.
You know you're Triple Negative,
Few options there to take!

And so you read the small print,
What was there, I damn near choked.
I couldn't get my head round it?
The order was a joke!

The side effects are listed,
So you'd think the worst was last.
But there it was, for number two,
It's Death! Well, what a blast!

Oh, the party carries on.
What a joy all this will be...
Sickness, baldness, diarrhoea,
Loss of.. fertility!?

And then vaginal dryness?
Oh now, that just took the piss!
All the menopausal symptoms?
I'm giving that a miss.

There's more, it just keeps going...
Other cancers, aches and pains.
Constipation, weight gain, sore mouth?
My soul lies down the drain.

Good god, it makes you wonder,
What the hell we do this for!?
And coz it all takes effing months,
To others.. we're a bore.

We do this coz we have to...
Yes, we want to bloody live!
So f**k them all! SE of C,
You won't hold me captive!

And if you ever wonder,
What this journey gave to me?
Just take some time and Google..
Chemotherapy SE.

Edwina Maria Thompson
© 2017

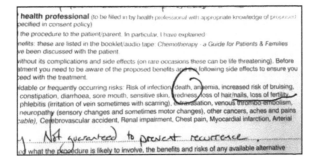

3rd October 2017

I've written this latest poem to salute the end of my treatments. It's a funny thing to call myself a TOAD, but it does make me giggle. (I even told Wendy- "If I die; I want everyone to change their profile picture on Facebook to a squashed toad." She wasn't amused at all, especially when I sent the pictures of squashed toads to her!) I've fallen on many occasions, yes; but the thing is... I always get back up. Even birds fall and if we don't fall once in a while; we will never learn and we will never grow.

A Toad On The Road

So here I am guys, Treatment Over And Done.
I'd book me a hol, if it's not in the sun.

A year I was told, from the rads the doc said?
So fragile my skin, but at least I'm not Dead...

That word, it's a smack! Such a slap in the face!
And Cancer and Chemo, not words we embrace.

Our treatment last months, and for some it takes years.
Then suddenly stops, leaving us with those fears...

We all have a choice. We can laugh, we can cry.
Our choice is to LIVE. Or sit waiting to die.

These lessons in life, are a chance to be taught.
So precious this life, not a thing to be bought.

My yoga I thought, is what taught me to love.
But cancer, your gifts, they spread far and above.

I've met special friends, by my side for all time.
Our angels we miss, but remember with wine!

It's all a new me, a new road to be tread.
Excited, impelled, I refuse to feel dread!

And yes, I will fall, but I focus on *TOAD*!
Treatment- Over- And- Done..
Get me back on that road!

Edwina Maria Thompson
© 2017

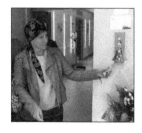

MOVING FORWARD

5th October 2017

Another fabulous meet up today with the warriors; there was Julie, Cath and I, but we were also joined by Louise Marie Preston. We met up at the Pet Place again so I could introduce Neo to Cath and Louise, and Julie brought Biddy with her. I'm pleased to say that they both got on very well. (Biddy and Neo I mean!) Julie brought this black hoof with her for Neo and a fleecy blanket for him to lie on; talk about being spoilt. She just can't resist those 'wayward' ears of his. I tell you what though, that hoof stank to high heaven, but god he loved it. It was quite busy today though, with lots of other dogs in; so we had plenty of attention from people. I can't deny it, we all do look like we are part of a club when we're together! It was a good way to get Triple Negative Breast Cancer known though as well and this has got to be my favourite picture of us all so far. I love it.

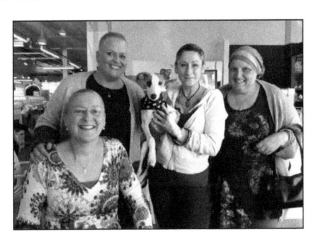

8ᵗʰ October 2017

Well, as usual, I decided I could run before I could walk .On Wednesday I saw the radiographer who told me to get back into my yoga gently, using my common sense. (Yeah, yeah I thought, I know.) On Friday, Julie and I went to the Moving Forward course. (This is a course run by Breast Cancer Care to help ladies find their feet again after breast cancer.) There was a nurse there to talk to us about lymphedema, (swelling in the arm when the lymphatic drainage isn't working correctly). I knew to avoid cuts, needles and the blood pressure monitor on your surgery side if any lymph nodes were taken. However, I had no idea about avoiding too much weight bearing!

I asked the question, what about yoga? I will be taking my whole body weight on my arms? Take your time she said, don't do an hour's class yet, build it up... (Oh shit I thought, I've tried 3 classes in the last 4 days! Whoops.) So what's happened to me after those 3 classes then? Well, yesterday was spent in bed all day, with both hands and arms numb most of the day. I was hardly able to stand let alone walk, and in complete agony all over! Today, I'm walking like a 90 year old, but I am walking! The moral of the story... listen to the experts and do as you're bloody well told! They clearly know what they're saying!

12ᵗʰ October 2017

This latest poem I have written may well cause controversy, so I'm preparing you. I get really wound up when people put cancer down to one cause; or pretty much blame your cancer on your own lifestyle. You can get cancer for a variety of reasons; particularly now they are looking to genetics. The latest 'cause' is sugar, in a year it will be something else. You can be the fittest, healthiest person and get cancer- (I was!) Those who think they can avoid all chances of developing

cancer by cutting out anything bad from their diets- are unbelievably naïve. 1 in 2 of us will get cancer, which is the sad fact
of the matter. We have been exposed to so much in our life-
times now, that we can run as far as we like: but we can't hide
from it. So I say everything in moderation, but with common
sense obviously. (I am not suggesting living on a diet of pizza,
coke, sweets and crisps either, now that is daft.) Just don't
deny yourself and enjoy life! I was at the peak of my health
and strength and still got cancer...

What's Next?

"It's sugar that caused this!" Oh god... now that's it?
Those "well meaning" know alls, who spout all their shit.

I wonder if ever they sit down and think?
How saying "You caused this...",
Takes us to the brink.

I was veggie, teetotal, vegan a while.
This body a temple, my "oms" with a smile.

But that didn't keep me from under the knife..
Coz frankly, my dear, that big 'C' is rife!

There's children and babies and pets for God's sake!
They all died from sugar? That theory's half baked.

So shove all your diets and shakes up your arse.
Coz hearing more 'causes', I'm watching a farce.

We're all in a club, WE DID NOT sign up for!
And saying we 'caused' it? That really is poor...

So off, you all trot, to prevent what you will.
Coz cancer is lurking and WILL have it's fill!

(And here's one for you, just in case I'm not clear.
I'll eat the damn cake, go add that to your rear!)

Edwina Maria Thompson
© 2017

13th October 2017

Wow! I am so excited! Julie sent me a post from the Christie Facebook page, where they are looking for poetry written by cancer patients and families. So I emailed them with a few of my poems, and I got a response. My poems are going into the World Mental Health Day booklet, I'm so made up!

14th October 2017

Not feeling too brill today, the radiotherapy fatigue is really beginning to take a hold. So as I don't have the energy to leave the house and visit friends; me and Julie just spent the day sending random pictures to each other instead! We definitely do love our little babies. (Babies, not dogs!)

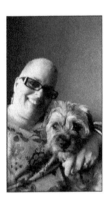 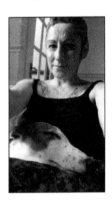

17th October 2017

I went right to the beginning of it all for this poem. I'd actually had a lump previously in January 2015 which was benign, but then another had appeared in 2016. This second one however, wasn't taken very seriously. Fast forward 8 months, and it had eventually been looked at more closely. After a month of being told my lump was 'unusual' and looked nothing like cancer, followed by ultrasounds, mammograms and biopsies, I finally went for my results. This was that day.

That Word You Fear

I sat and waited, head hung low.
My instincts sighed, it's 'yes' you know.
I looked around, this place was bare.
No place to learn, life wasn't fair.
I'd been before, nothing amiss.
A different room, so unlike this.
These walls were grey, no comfy chair.
Perched on a bed, no softness there...

My journey here, had took so long.
All year I sensed, so much was wrong.
The visits back and forth in vain,
More bloods and samples, sweats and pains.
My body cried, what's going on?
Just get it out, or you're long gone!
My mind returned, the doc flew in.
His tie askew, a smile to win...

"How can I help?"
An air of cheer?
So did this mean, results were clear?
"You sent for me?", my voice unsure.
"Oh right, I see"... back out the door.
Hushed voices heard, a rush for notes.
Door softly shut, and with it, hopes.
It felt by now, just like my dreams.
Nothing prepares, what cancer means...

He swept back in, the cheer now lost.
Aware of what his slip had cost.
"Oh yes", he said, "Results are here.
It's Cancer, yes "... that word you fear.
He's got it wrong, my doubt was high.
It just can't be my time to die?
"You've been before, benign I see.
In Jan '15?"

Oh god, that's me...

You can't imagine, how it feels,
You mind goes numb, heart at your heels.
The floor just starts to fall away,
Your mouth is dry, your feet like clay.
As notes recite the fight you face.
The walls close in, no breathing space.
They say you never hear a word.
Take someone close, so steps are heard...

I turned to him, I held his hand.
This wasn't quite what we had planned.
I knew, I saw, he'd never leave.
He'd be my air, he'd help me breathe.
It felt right then, my fight was won.
Coz love gives hope, all said and done.
And so we left, my hopes felt high.

I'm right, it's not my time to die.

Edwina Maria Thompson
© 2017

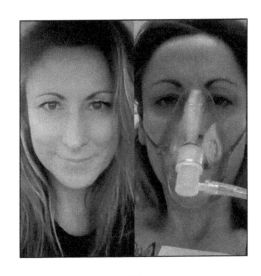

72

17th October 2017

When I wrote 'Who Am I?' I never envisaged a point where I would be happy to look into the mirror again. It felt like a lifetime while I was wearing wigs or scarves, drawing on eyebrows and filling in with eyeliner. But here I am, less than 3 months later, and I am finding myself again! This is the sister poem to Who Am I? and this to me proves that despite everything: that phoenix will arise. I will always have my wolf female spirit, and of course, my warrior of old. I promise you, it really does return.

A Phoenix, A Wolf,
A Warrior, And Me.

I look in the mirror
And what do I see.
A phoenix arising
From ashes of me.

I look at these eyes,
Truly bright and they shine.
My eyebrows, so dark now,
And guess what, they're mine!

With hair like a pixie,
All black, grey and white.
My God, how it's diff'rent!
A beautiful sight!

My skin so fresh faced,
With a head full of curls.
I'm already planning,
Night's out with the girls.

They said it grows back...
Just too hard to believe.
The waiting is endless.
Your image... you grieve.

But time passes by.
As you're yearning for 'you',
And what will appear is,
Somebody brand new!

A fighter will grow,
As the battles are drawn,
I promise, she's in there,
A warrior's born!

So next time you see me,
Look right in my face.
This girl holds no punches,
A wolf took her place!

I looked in the mirror,
This morning to see.
A phoenix, a wolf and
A warrior... all me!

Edwina Maria Thompson
© 2017

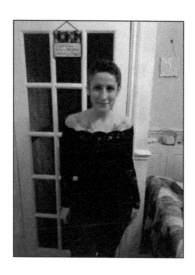

20th October 2017

I met a lovely lady recently on the Moving Forward Course who inspired me to write this. She had just had a beautiful little girl, then she was diagnosed with cancer. The emotion she had experienced beyond anything else- was anger. Anger that this could happen to her at what should have been the happiest time of her life; anger at how ruthless cancer is. A few weeks ago, Julie, Emma and I stood in the car park, talking about how unfair Triple Negative is. How cruel that it targeted such young women; young mothers and in some cases, women who hadn't even had the opportunity to have children if they wished. I drove home that day, repeating her words in my head... "IT'S NOT FAIR!" She is so right, it's not fair and we have every right to be angry by it.

I write an edit to this as I put everything together. In truth, this poem wasn't just for Emma; it was also for Julie and I. We would often speak about our children having to cope with us having cancer. We were all too aware, age didn't matter when it came to the love we had for them, and theirs for us. We wanted to see them grow into adults, to see them marry possibly and to have children of their own. Why shouldn't we? So when I wrote this, the last verses were actually for all three of us- Emma, Julie and me, and of course, for all of our children. Thank you also to Emma for the beautiful picture!

IT'S NOT FAIR!

"IT'S NOT FAIR, I'M FUCKING MAD!!"
I'll scream until I'm hoarse.
Don't question that I'm angry,
Please let it run its course.

I don't want bloody 'wings' yet,
Or memories to be shared.
I want to hold my baby,
When she's lonely or she's scared.

She smiles at me so trusting,
I'll always be right there.
That that may never happen...
Tell me how that is FAIR!?

I'm gazing at her fingers,
And kissing tiny toes.
The love and bond between us,
With every moment grows.

I gave birth to my angel,
Then found this shit disease!
A fucking EVIL BASTARD!
What God would do this, please?

I'd say "Excuse my language."
But guess what, I don't care!
A mother with a baby?!
IT'S JUST NOT FUCKING FAIR!

I want to watch her grow up,
To walk and talk and play.
To see her bright eyes light up,
In school for her first day.

Excitement when it's Christmas!
The first time she sees snow,
And finding gifts from Santa,
That precious smile aglow.

Then what about her future?
A bride in white one day?
To have those times without me?
With breaking heart, I pray.

A mother shouldn't have to,
Think devastating words,
"My time with you is fading."
It's totally absurd!

We want to raise our children,
No shit to hit the fan.
We will NOT break their sweet hearts,
But be the best we can.

And so we beg for those years,
A natural decrease...
Please God just get us through this,
Pray, let us live in peace.

Edwina Maria Thompson
© 2017

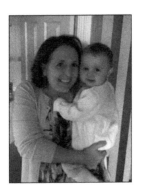

21st October 2017

Wow! My poetry is now in the Christie World Mental Health Day booklet. How utterly amazing is that. I never in a million years thought that cancer would lead me to having poetry published. There are 3 of them in there; I am so utterly excited! God I love life and what it brings when you least expect it. It never ever ceases to amaze me.

23rd October 2017
The Warrior Rising

Well this week is the start of me dipping my toes back into some classes. I'll be totally honest, (as you've got used to now), I'm not up to much. I look great, but the body is shit. This is all from side effects of chemotherapy, which may stay or pass: but for now are massively holding me back on my mat. That I might add just means I won't demonstrate much. I actually think this is a good thing, I won't be teaching flowing poses from one to the next one, building up that sweat. I will be slowing things right down: 'stir sukhan asanan', which is 'steady and comfortable, pose' of course. We spend enough of our time racing around from one job to the next, keeping it all going 'just right'... so maybe it's time to slow down on our mats too.

I'm not bothered if I ever have the ability to do a handstand or headstand ever again in my own practise. Yoga was never about the poses, it was about me feeling alive and free! So what if my current standard is at a beginner's level, being there is teaching me more than you can ever imagine. For a while there, getting on my mat was just reminding me of what I couldn't do, how much I'd changed. My ego was massively bruised, and I knew it. It took some serious looking inwards to see what good was coming from all of this. But I did, and

I know there are great things to come. For now, I'll leave you with the skill I have acquired from all this crap, writing poems. Yoga I guess still... just under a different guise.

So, this new one is the sister poem to S.E. of C. It started in my head a few nights back, when I was throwing the covers on and off all night trying to cool down. My leg was in and out of the covers constantly! Unfortunately, one of the many gifts of chemotherapy, (especially if you are of a certain age) is the menopause. Now I'll be honest, I wasn't bothered by this at all. My kids are grown up now, and I have NO intention of having any more. However, TN is more common in ladies under 40 years of age, so this side effect can be utterly devastating for them. In some cases, their only course of action is to have their eggs frozen and hope. This poem is very much for them.

Menopause and Me

So getting back to menopause,
From chemotherapy.
I'm lucky coz I'm 48,
I've had my family.

I do NOT mind the loss of blood,
I'm sorry to be frank.
Coz mopping up for 30 years,
Was pretty bloody rank!

But suddenly I have these waves,
Hot flushes in the day.
Get windows open, sod the cold,
Just give me breeze I pray!

They even come when you're asleep,
Hot sweats that drive you mad.
You wake up in a puddle, soaked!
What games there, to be had...

Leg in, leg out, leg in, leg out,
It makes you scream and shout.
The hokey cokey in your bed,
Is not what it's about!

And then an angry Hulk appears,
A mood swing in a flash!
God help all those, who cross you now...
No anger seems too rash!

The bright sparks always have their say,
"Of course, you're getting old..."
It's chemotherapy not age,
Won't you be bloody told!?

You see, I might make light of this,
With what the chemo's done.
And let you all, just have a laugh...
Coz then it feels like fun.

So no more jokes, bring thoughts to these,
The ladies who are young.
They may have wanted children yet...
So chemo's really stung.

This f**ked cancer I have had,
TNBC, it's name.
It targets more the younger ones,
To 40, that's NO game.

They really have no options there,
As hormones are no use.
It's chemo, rads, with all the risk
Of side effects abuse.

So send your love and prayers to them...
Young women in this boat.
That menopause will steer them by,
Their dreams to stay afloat.

Edwina Maria Thompson
© 2017

24th October 2017

This is a poem I've had great fun writing. I definitely did feel like I was radioactive after going to the nuclear department in the hospital! It took me a while to get this one right though, and I had a lot of help from Julie. I must have sent it to her a few times until she said it flowed correctly. She is my muse! (Her favourite lines are 'Woo Hoo I'm kryptonite' and 'my blue tit'!) Statistics do say now that 1 in 2 of us will develop some sort of cancer in our lives. Not the best of odds is it, a little like tossing a coin. So we best feel grateful for everything we have and never ever forget that!

The 50/50 Club

So here I am, all signed up to...
A club I didn't join.
50/50
Cancer odds.
I could have tossed a coin!

Your surgeon tells you what's ahead,
But really, you've no clue.
I think he said,
First surgery,
Then something about blue?

The blue bit didn't make much sense,
But now I know too well.
My 'Blue tit' shows,
He checked lymph nodes
Were free of cancer cells.

Injected in the breast with dye.
To travel through my nodes.
Geiger counter,
Used to find
First ones, and what they showed.

So now I'm radioactive, yey!!
Woo hoo, I'm kryptonite!
Whoops, sorry there,
I lost myself...
You gotta laugh alright!

I've never seen an advert say,
How many types there are.
It's just a lump?
So cut it out!
How easy's that... so far?

Specifics come with your report,
It's Triple Negative?
Dr. Google
Straight away,
You what? Less chance to live!

In breast cancer, it is quite rare,
Stats say, 15 percent.
Then genes may have,
Mutations from
Your family descent.

And just to top it off for you,
It's usually grade 3,
Aggressive with
It's nature, in
Breast cancer family.

No hormones in it's make up, with
No long term treatment there.
Only chemo
And the rads,
It doesn't seem quite fair.

The chances of recurrence, and
The spread is higher too.
Yes, Google tolls
A bell so clear...
The short straw there you drew!

You turn into an expert on,
The term 'TNBC'.
Ask any Question,
We may know.
We could take a degree!

More common in young ladies of,
They say, 40 or less.
It's so unfair,
They have to bear
These odds and such distress.

It really is that scary, though
Our future is unknown.
Once treatment's done,
The great abyss,
Is where you feel you're thrown.

But, here I am, signed off and done,
No more 'TNBC'.
I'm in the 'club',
But I have won,
A whole new family.

For now we all are warriors,
In unity we stand.
No matter what,
Lies far ahead,
We'll face it hand in hand.

Edwina Maria Thompson
© 2017

25th October 2017

During my treatment, I made a pretty huge decision... I wanted a puppy. I'd wanted a dog for years, but life was always too busy. I even sat down one day, working out how many hours I would be out at a time; so my virtual dog wouldn't be in their cage too long. Then cancer came into my life, and made me say; sod it, get me that puppy! He is a godsend to me now, and it is probably the best thing I could have ever done. He has changed my life completely. This one is for my adorable pup Neo, his name chosen for it's meaning.... new. (His name is also a nod to the character of 'Neo' in the film The Matrix, who is referred to as 'The One'.)

The 'One'

"Life's just too short", my mind's made up.
"Now treatment's done, I'll buy a pup."
I knew that some, would think me mad,
But let them have, the year I'd had!

I went through different types of breed,
To find the one to suit my needs.
A little daft, a little wild,
But loving, with a temper mild.

Decision made, a whippet dog,
A couch potato, sofa hog!
I knew he would, like Velcro stick,
And as for 'walkies', he'd be quick!

I Googled adverts, searching for,
The perfect puppy, I'd adore.
It wasn't long before I found,
Cute furry babies, bellies round.

One face stood out, with open jaw.
All playful mischief that I saw!
My instinct kicked in, "He's 'The One'."
Let him be there, not sold and gone.

The very first time that we met,
Is not a thing I will forget.
They say the right one, comes to you...
Our little pup, he nearly flew!

His siblings round, a push right through.
That he was ours, I'm sure he knew!
Up on hind legs, he tried to stand.
With cold wet nose, sniff of my hand.

Those big blue eyes, a cheeky look,
My heart just melted, I was hooked!
Deposit paid, (we weren't too late),
But 5 more weeks we had to wait.

The day it came, for us to go,
And bring back home, our pet 'Neo'.
It even seemed, the calendar,
Knew this.. 'A day to remember'.

Our precious puppy has a goal,
A healing for heart, mind and soul.
Right by my side, both night and day,
To keep that 'ticking bomb' at bay.

And those who doubt, he's therapy.
Just see the joy, he brings to me.
That smile lights up, my face and eyes.
He's always there, through lows and highs.

'A new beginning', he has brought.
The perfect prize, for battles fought.
So now I'll put back down my pen,
And cuddle Neo once again.

Edwina Maria Thompson
© 2017

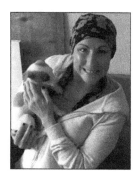

26th October 2017

Today I was talking to Julie and another lady on the Moving Forward course. I was very amused to hear things a mastectomy boob is used for: rather than it's actual job! Emma's little girl shoves it under her top and says 'baby', and Julie's son put hers on his head. Absolutely hilarious, I love it! I think I feel a poem coming on...

27th October 2017

This poem has been inspired by my breast cancer nurse Elizabeth. I went to see her a few days ago as I'm really struggling with the whole 'end of treatment' thing; and ended up in tears in her room. So she reminded me of what I've been through, that basically I've been expecting far too much of myself recently. She said to me, "Don't forget, you have been cut, poisoned and burned." It struck me as quite horrific when she put it that way, but effectively, that IS what has been done to us. We do have to remember, it is a hugely traumatic experience we have gone through. So thank you for that little reminder Elizabeth. Surgery- cut; chemotherapy- poisoned and radiotherapy- burned. My god, that actually sounds like torture.

Surgery, Chemo and Rads.

'Cut, poisoned and burned.'
A term,
Grudgingly learned.
As treatment I know,
Of cancer may go,
With
Cut, poisoned and burned.

Cut, poisoned and burned.
Our minds,
Frantically churned.
No advert will show,
The truth of this foe.
We're
Cut, poisoned and burned.

Cut, poisoned and burned.
The lump,
Surgeon has spurned.
My breast now hollow,
A scar to follow.
I'm
Cut, poisoned and burned.

Cut, poisoned and burned.
Respect,
This I have earned!
Shot up with chemo,
Then body aglow.
All
Cut, poisoned and burned.

Cut, poisoned and burned.
Survived,
Body returned!

My hair I forego,
But back it will grow
From
Cut, poisoned and burned.

Cut, poisoned and burned.
Relief,
I am adjourned.
But prayers I bestow ,
To those in the flow
Of
Cut, poisoned and burned.

Edwina Maria Thompson
© 2017

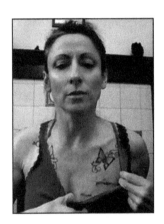
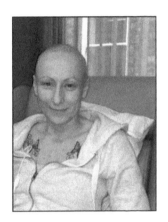
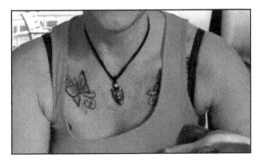

THE BLACK DOG

29th October 2017

When you come to the end of cancer treatment, they say it can be a more difficult time than the treatment itself. Even though you know how lucky you are- many suffer similar symptoms to PTSD. Having suffered from depression in the past, I am anticipating this... so I've bought a puppy Neo to help me through that time. He is the best therapy ever!

This poem comes from the conversations I've been having with Julie at the Moving Forward course. We both keep waking up in the middle of the night, worrying and wondering if our cancer will ever return or if it has spread. I always look to my phone to see if Julie is awake too. I liken it to holding a Time Bomb, not sure whether it will ever go off, but still having to listen to that 'tick, tick, tick'. At night time of course, it is a lot louder. Julie was saying that her nurse describes Cancer as being 'right up in your face' and that you can't see around it. All you can see is the cancer. Somehow you have to find a way to pull it back so it's not all consuming; but this is considerably easier said than done. As our cancer is Triple Negative, we aren't offered any long term medication after treatment. There isn't anything to give us. We just have to hope over the coming 5 years, that our cancer has gone for good.

Nothing prepares you for this aftermath, even though you know it's coming. You can only batten down the hatches and pray.

Tick Tock

So here I am awake at night,
My thoughts becoming dark.
The future, now unclear to me...
So fearful, haunting, stark.
A ticking bomb, my weight to bear,
That may NEVER explode.
It's ticking soft I find by day;
At night, a heavy load.

It's ticking grows with every dread,
This scourge, it may return.
The fear that once again you'll face,
More cuts and poisons, burns.
A sentence of 5 years I hold,
A jailor none can see.
That ticking bomb reminding me,
I'm done; but far from free.

As final days approach from months,
Of treatments you endure.
The hopes and prayers they rest that now...
You won't need anymore
Anticipation teases of,
A desperate stay from death.
No quelling of the ticking bomb,
Just counting every breath.

That bomb, I now will place aside,
To aid my sanity.
But darker humour does desire,
The odd profanity.
So f**k my bomb, it's ticking doom,
May never it ignite..
No way will you my spirit break!
This girl retained her fight!

Edwina Maria Thompson
© 2017

92

29th October 2017

I waited today at The Christie in Wigan to make an appointment. An elderly lady came and stood next to me, and my whole being suddenly felt devastated. She had clearly just had the worst news, and I could feel it. Her friend was holding her hand and the old lady whispered, 'I just want to go home'. I genuinely wanted to cry for her, her pain felt so overwhelming. I don't know who she was, but it made me think of those older couples; those who have been with their loved one all of their lives. It reminded me of the story my mother told me about my Great Grandparents. How when my Great Grandma died, my Great Granddad died only weeks later; he literally just gave up. He couldn't bear to be without her. It must be utterly heart- breaking when one half of an elderly couple dies, leaving the other one heartbroken and alone.

The Eulogy

The time had come. His gaze now fell,
to take a moment's thought.
No length of time prepared him for,
the grief his loss had brought.
With bitter hopelessness,
their final weeks had slowly crept.
Grave memories of holding tight,
a veil of tears they'd wept.

"She was my world"... no more to say;
beyond that, he was void.
To see her twinkling eyes erased,
his shattered heart destroyed.
Quite where to start this life
again- there was no hope but dread.
Their smiles and laughter,
left behind... an emptiness ahead.

Then patient hushes roused his thoughts,
from tender looks around.
No hiding from this fated task, inevitably bound.
Beside the casket, hollow gait, a shadow of the man.
A shaking voice, a gentle touch, "I'll do the best I can."

"We met so young." His jaded tones,
"And fell in love, first sight.
Every single day we had, I'd kiss and squeeze her tight.
We married within four short months,
the perfect bride for me.
And blessed we've been, for we have had, a happy family."

"I come to you, a broken man,
who watched his sweetheart die.
And rather would I go with her, I cannot tell a lie.
I miss each day, her smiling face; her quirky little grin.
With dignity, she fought for life; such pain in death, a sin."

"Not once did she complain throughout her chemotherapy.
The sickness, needles, suffering... she bore them all for me."
A pause for air, to catch a breath, the sorrow all too great.
His tears, like a waterfall, a river could create.

Then closing eyes, he felt her reach,
to stroke an anguished brow.
Her whispers gentle in his ear, "Just hang on in, for now."
But little more that he could say, too much was his heartache.
A moment to compose himself, for effort must he make.

"For 60 years she was my wife, my best friend and my guide.
I am bereft and set adrift, without her by my side.
The overwhelming love she gave, it made of me, a king.
She was my life, my universe, my girl, my everything."

As final words had left dry lips, he faltered in the aisle.
Then memories of golden times, brought flickers of a smile.
A daughter kindly took his hand, and led him to their place.
And so they sat, both gathered in, their angel's soft embrace.

Edwina Maria Thompson
© 2017

30ᵗʰ October 2017

My yoga mat has been my place of safety now for 6 years. It has been the place where I rebuilt my confidence and found my strength mentally, physically and emotionally; where I began to believe in myself again. It has been both my saviour and my guide on so many occasions.

I remember standing once in a pose once called 'Dancer's pose' or 'Nataranjasana'. This involved me standing on one leg, reaching behind to catch hold of my foot and balancing in a beautiful, graceful and balletic way. Yet while I was in that pose, the tears were streaming down my face with heartbreak and hurt. Another time, I was in a 'yogic' headstand, again with tears streaming down my face soaking into my hair. Even at my worst times I would stand in a warrior pose with my feet gripped to the earth, telling myself, no matter how many times the rug was ripped from beneath my feet- I would always stand tall and strong!

Each and every time, I was able to control my thoughts, because I had the poses to give me my fight and hope. I was thinking: 'Throw anything at me- I can live through it and learn from it. You cannot break me- I will always still be able to stand on my head!' Now here I am: I can neither stand on my head nor balance with ease. My body has never felt as broken as it does now; I am desperately trying to figure this out. I am lost completely and utterly. What is my lesson here? What is my purpose if I can no longer roll out my mat with hope? What am I meant to do now? If I can't do yoga, what do I do?

<u>Drifting</u>

It's hard to explain, to say how I feel.
And sometimes it's like, not one thing is real.

When I felt adrift, I'd roll out my mat.
My place to escape; some peace while I sat.

In poses I found, my soul was reborn.
This heart would ignite, so sweetly untorn.

A refuge, my mat, the place I would go.
To find some more fight, and handle each show.

But now there it lies, futile in my room.
It watches and waits, an omen of doom.

A battle it brings, that I must endure.
The poses I find, no longer my cure.

This warrior's lost, her ultimate pose.
I have little strength, my failure, it grows.

Two voices I hear, so clear in my mind.
A wretched one grim... Thank God one is kind.

The wretched one sighs, "You'll never feel right.
Coz each time you'll fail... regardless of fight."

The kind voice inspires, she says "It's Ok.
You cry all your tears, it's just 'Hippo' day."

"Go wallow and sink, roll round in the mud.
Accept that things change, but life is still good."

"Let all of it out, and scream if you need.
Yes, life just got tough... but it sows a seed."

97

I'll not be the same, and that I accept.
A new 'me' will rise, from tears that I wept.

The drifting will end, I'll stand tall and strong.
My warrior was... right there, all along.

Edwina Maria Thompson
© 2017

1st November 2017

I know I am on this journey and that it is like the 'Road to Hell' at times; but so far, I am lucky in all of this: I haven't been given a terminal diagnosis, as so many have been. I was speaking to a lovely lady recently, who had lost her brother to cancer. He hadn't told his family how long he had, or how bad his prognosis was. She described him as the most incredible, inspiring and beautiful man. Knowing he didn't have long, he had begun to leave 'post it' notes around the house; with little messages for his family.

I found this so kind and selfless: worrying about your family's well-being, after you have gone. I think that it is the thing we all worry about the most. I began to imagine what would have happened, had it been me going through this journey; but when my children were young. I was also reminded of the programme about Rio Ferdinand earlier this year, and how his wife had passed away with young children. The memory jar they created after her death was so touching; and it made me wonder if I would have thought to make one too.

Many years ago, I told my friend Vannessa that I was going to write a letter to my daughters every year: letters of our memories, my thoughts and possibly some advice in life. This was long before cancer came. I sensed that it was important to leave a little something of me behind for them, just in case. Yet I never did it, I was always too busy. I guess now that my poems and blogs have become that 'little something', so I do have a legacy to leave. Hopefully, it will be me they'll get to keep for many years though and not my words.

This is for all of those women and men raising children young or old. My thoughts and prayers go to you every day.

No More Time

Those fateful words hung in the air,
"You're now on borrowed time."
No shock she felt, no huge despair,
No death bell or it's chime.
Of all the things her thoughts to be...
She'd better write a list...
God help them sorting out the house,
It's then that she'd be missed!

The journey home, they carried on,
With conversations dull.
Much easier to focus on,
The drab and trivial.
But really they were skirting past,
The horror on their minds.
The best way now, to break the news,
To which they were resigned.

Where do you start to tell your kids?
"Your Mummy's gonna die..."
And find an answer, they'll accept,
To when they question "Why?"
She couldn't justify their loss,
And racked her head in vain.
It felt right now, a living hell;
That she would cause their pain.

Her job should be to hold them tight,
And kiss their tears away,
To take their hands and let them know,
That everything's ok.
To have some fun and silliness,
Coz childhood goes so fast.
Why should they think or have that fear...
"Is this day Mummy's last?"

Her thoughts again returned to all,
The little things she did.
No time to waste, get on that list,
Stop being so morbid!
Jot down their favourite songs and games,
Which TV channel's best,
And how to always keep your cool,
When you're put to the test!

She thought to make a special box,
Of precious times to keep.
Some photographs and memories,
To make them smile, not weep.
The time when Zoe hid the keys,
And tripped her down the stairs!
How Robin used to love those books,
Of fairies, wolves and bears.

The many holidays they took,
To Lapland, Greece and Spain.
Them climbing up Egyptian hills,
In dusty, hot terrain!
Each memory would hold a note,
Her words of love to them.
At 18, theirs to open up,
Remembering again...

Back to her list and household stuff...
(She still did the most part!)
Post-it notes she'd leave in place so,
He'd know where to start...
The thought of leaving him behind,
To mop up from this mess.
He'd been her rock, her saviour through,
This un-ending distress.

His world ahead, a widower,
A single dad, so young!
She hoped his friends delivered with,
The promises they'd sung.
Of course there were some places he,
Could go for 'grief support'.
That's more things for her growing list,
'Help' numbers she could sort!

Why hadn't this occurred before?
This list would take all year!
And not predicted "weeks or months",
Those words so crystal clear...
It's funny how she looked so well,
There's not a soul would know;
That there was she, that ticking bomb,
All primed and set to blow.

Edwina Maria Thompson
© 2017

2nd November 2017

Cancer has touched us a few times in my family; with aunties and uncles who have passed away from this disease. My Uncle John had died of prostate cancer in October of 2016, only a matter of months before my own diagnosis. He was a priest, a truly special soul and an absolute inspiration to everyone who ever met him. In his last days, I visited and sang a mantra to him (he loved Sanskrit chanting). It was haunting the way the sounds filled the room, nearly bringing my mother to tears. What made it even more incredible was that he joined in with me; he sang words that he couldn't possibly have known. My mother, my Uncle Michael and I were astounded- it felt like we had just witnessed a miracle of some sort. Ironically, I realise now: as he was coming to the last days of his cancer journey, I was about to begin my own. Maybe that was why those words had such a powerful effect on us all.

After I'd had my cancer diagnosis however, my first thought of all things was... 'Get me to Costa'. (Talk about getting your priorities right!) I think, looking back, it was the normality of the place I needed. I know phoning my daughters to tell them I had cancer, was not the best way to break the news. So hopefully I've made it up to them now. This poem follows on from 'That Word You Fear', it tells of what happened next...

COSTA Then Kids

"What now?" I thought, "Do we go home,
And make a list of who to phone?"
My news, let's face it, was the worst.
"Prioritise! What should come first?"
Sat in the car, it felt surreal.
My world now turned, head over heels.
"What do you need?" My partner's voice,
"Just take a moment, it's your choice."

"A COSTA coffee, caffeine fix!
And throw some chocolate in the mix."
To COSTA first? That felt quite mean.
But coffee helped, cohere this dream...
"A latte please, with caramel.
It might just wake me from this hell.
We need to sit and think this through.
My mind is lost, with what to do."

My girls came first, now that was clear.
In simple terms, DO NOT cause fear.
Oh God, then Mum. What do I say?
Her brother John, just passed away.
A Holy man, his death so wrong.
This same disease, he fought too long.
I knew no matter what I said,
She'd worry sick, and think me dead...

The one thing that I knew for sure,
I must make light, and reassure.
Just let them know, I was ok.
And planned to fight it, all the way!
My coffee gone, the time had come,
To phone my girls, and then my mum.
I couldn't handle, face to face,
For now, I needed breathing space...

The first call was, so hard to make,
"It's cancer"... that's SHIT news to break.
I wrapped it up and kept it short,
A phone call's best, or so I thought...
It seemed they both, were really calm,
Considering, I'd dropped a bomb.
I promised I would come to theirs,
To let them know the 'how's' and 'where's'.

The next to come, a harder call.
With cancer's strike, now me to fall.
In my mum's eyes, I was the last.
Her 'baby' still, though decades passed.
For her sake, I would play it down.
(That C word wears Grim Reaper's gown.)
I told her straight, it's cancer, yes...
Don't worry please, and don't obsess!

Back then, I thought it better to,
Not make a fuss, and just make do.
I told them all, "They'll cut it out,
But chemo, NO. Of that, no doubt."
In time I found, once weeks had gone.
At twenty two, and twenty one,
How bad my girls' anxiety,
That I might die. Their mother.
Me.

So came a day, a nurse had said,
My cancer was a type to spread.
The treatment was a shock to see,
6 rounds of chemotherapy...
I made my choice, "Where do I sign?"
I'd do it for, these girls of mine.
They needed me, to know I care,
Enough to even lose my hair...

I'd take the rads, I'd take the scars.
For them, I'd fly from Earth to Mars.
There's nothing that I wouldn't do,
For them and me, I'd make it through.
So now I'm here! The other side!
My hair's grown back, no need to hide.
And if my cancer comes again,
It's COSTA first, then fight for them.

Edwina Maria Thompson
© 2017

5th November 2017

Well everyone... I am finally putting my poems out there for you all to share! There is a Facebook page I have created now called A Warrior's Words (maybe I'll even write a book one day.) This way if you know anyone touched by cancer and would like a voice for how cancer feels- you can head this way. Please do let your friends and families know as I'm finding they are very therapeutic and touch many people. So many of us are affected by cancer now, and these might just help a little.

6th November 2017

Julie told me about a new website, (I told you she is my muse!) It is called the Breast Cancer Art Project and has been founded by a lovely lady called Adriana. She only began this project in October 2017 and there have already been loads of contributions to it! You will find art work, poetry, photography, and I have a poem in there too now. How amazing is that, I am on the Internet with poetry. As Julie has said to me- "Poetry world domination!"

19th November 2017

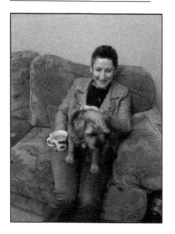

I've been to visit Julie today at her home. She has had the most devastating news- that her cancer has spread. The boils on her skin she has been suffering from, aren't boils- they're cancer. It is beyond me that this could happen to Julie of all people. My heart breaks for her and her family. It is completely f**king unfair. Her bravery is so incredible though and if I know Julie, she'll fight like hell! There was a lot we chatted about, but she will have to wait to see what the next steps are. A different chemo is what they will probably do and I hope to god it works this time. It has to. We know that the EC and Paclitaxol haven't worked so far and that is what is so cruel about TN, it is an absolute bastard with many ladies.

There just seems to be no rhyme or reason as to why it works with some and not others. We spoke about the protein called KI67 that was in our tumours. It is this that is used to grade the cancer (so we believe anyway) and anything above 20% is Grade 3, the most aggressive. (Most Triple Negative tumours are aggressive.) The higher the percentage is, the more aggressive the cancer. However, the more effective the chemotherapy then is. It's a catch 22, you just can't win. Do you want a cancer that is more sensitive to chemo or one that grows slowly and may be less sensitive? (Then of course, the metastatic tumours can have a different percentage to the primary tumour, so a prognosis can be difficult to determine.) The whole thing is a minefield!

I know she will need all of the warriors love and support more than ever now. I said anything she needed, she was just to shout! It was lovely to sit and play with Biddy too; I definitely think I have found a friend.

20th November 2017

There are many different types of cancers out there, all cruel and heart breaking. Personally, I don't like to say that one is 'worse' or 'easier' than another, we are all broken by cancer in some way. You do find yourself drawn however, to those with the same type as you. I am Triple Negative Breast Cancer of course, and my journey has led me to the most incredible group of women. So when one of us gets the worst news- we are all devastated by this. We are warriors, we are sisters, we are a family and we stand together as one.

This poem is for one special lady I love dearly- Julie, who has been given the news we dread the most; but it is also for everyone out there facing down this battle with TNBC. All of my love and prayers go now to Julie to help her in her battle with this piece of evil shit. I wrote this shortly after she phoned me to give me the news. As I drove to teach my yoga class, I was screaming it in my head- 'We are all in front of a fucking firing squad and we will fight to the death!'

<u>Firing Squad</u>

You stand before a firing squad,
Just waiting for that sound.
Each one of you has been shot once,
But there are still more rounds.
There is no rhyme nor reason to,
Which person will be hit.
But standing in that firing line,
Is really fucking SHIT!

You've no idea who is next,
As he chose randomly.
You're mothers, sisters, daughters, wives,
But that won't set you free.
It doesn't matter who is shot,
Because you have all grown,
To love the people nearest you,
As sisters you have known.

All warriors have different scars,
As some were shot so close.
The stronger ones stand ready with
Their arrows and their bows.
They know defense is grueling but,
They never will stand down!
That EVIL BASTARD with the gun,
Still thinks he owns this town!

You know that he is merciless,
With final shots to come.
But you have faced this foe before,
Like hell will you succumb!
You stand in line with hands held tight,
All ready to support,
The warriors that take a shot...
As one that battles fought.

I swear to god, each shot he takes,
It makes our spirits soar.
There is no way we will give up,
Just hear our Tribal roar!
So take your fucking senseless gun,
Coz Cancer you have picked,
The toughest band of warriors,
And your arse will be kicked!

Edwina Maria Thompson
© 2017

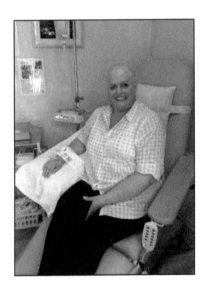

26th November 2017

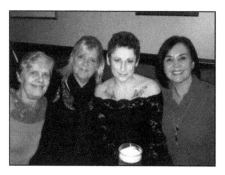

I held a 'Thanksgiving Party' on Friday night to thank all my students and friends for their love, help and support over the year. (Absolutely nothing to do with the American celebration though, I just pinched the name.) The amount of people who came was wonderful, and the pasties went down a treat! It was the first time in photos since January that I didn't look like the one who'd had cancer. How fabulous is that eh? It was the best time I have had in ages and we danced late into the night: it couldn't have been better.

There was one very special lady there that I wanted to give my thanks to more than most, Wendy. She has been my voice of reason, my guru (she'll kill me for that one) and the one who has had my back throughout. Ironically, Wendy was once my yoga student, and it was I who helped her. Now the tide has turned and the student becomes the teacher. What an intricate web this universe weaves for us and this is just how life should be, each of us 'paying it forward'. This is my little gift to her. Wendy, you mean the world to me and so I thank you from the bottom of my heart.

Virabhadra, (A Hero Friend)

When I first met Wendy,
She wasn't her best.
To put it quite bluntly,
She needed a rest!
Her job as a teacher,
Was draining her soul.
I knew of that darkness...
A black hellish hole.

My past mirrored in her,
I knew what to do.
Yoga, pranayama.
Of course, mantra too!
I watched as the weeks passed,
To see how she coped.
Ganesha might free her,
Is what I had hoped.

One lesson that really,
Just sticks in my mind.
Her chakras to balance,
To calm and unwind.
It seemed to just touch her,
And add to this flow
Of changes in motion.
All helping her grow.

She made a decision,
India! she'd fly.
The ashram to train there,
And reach for the sky!
It left an impression,
I know, from the start.
That sounding of 'AUM' now,
Resides in her heart.

She soon took on classes,
Instructing, like me.
To pay it all forward,
A true yogini.
As many years passed by,
More changes took root,
With pregnancy yoga,
Then Uni to boot!

This woman astounds me,
A spirit unbound.
But more we had coming,
So much more, I found.
A bomb shell dropped on me,
A shock, nothing less.
To share diagnosis,
Not fun, I confess.

For cancer had crossed her,
I knew... many ways.
To tell her, "And me too"
We'd had better days.
I tried to make light but,
This girl saw right through.
Her turn to help me now,
She knew what to do.

She gathered the tribe round,
To cushion my fall.
The warriors rushed to,
The sound of her call.
In school by the day time,
My classes by night!
She took away worry,
As I fought my fight.

She's my voice of reason,
Not scared to be harsh.
She tells me, "Go Easy!"
(My kick up the arse.)
"Your cycle of grieving,
You must give it time.
But not to consume you,
Or harder the climb."

She says toxic feelings,
Will not make things right.
"Ditch anger, guilt, sorrow,
And channel your fight."
Quite where I begin now,
To thank her, God knows!
I guess this is my way,
Through party and prose.

A mother, wife, daughter,
Sister.. 'Hero Friend.'
A Warrior unique!
Your kindness, no end.
So thanks to you Wendy,
Quite simply... a star.
Go shine ever brightly.
Guide those, near and far.

Edwina Maria Thompson
© 2017

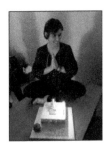

2nd December 2017

Ground Zero

I've thought long and hard as to whether I should be completely open to you all- whether I should tell you where I have found myself now. Throughout this journey I have been honest, brutal, and raw. I have let you know exactly what I am learning, feeling and experiencing. I'm guessing none of you have been surprised at what I've said over this year, cancer and it's treatment are a big deal. I have faced that mountain, all the shit it threw at me and I have climbed it. I've got the scars, pains and traumas to show for it. I won, it would seem. So is that now the end? No.

Throughout treatment I had a focus, something to do. It is common after treatment to hit a brick wall, similar to PTSD. I haven't hit a wall; I've opened my eyes to see another bloody mountain. Just as hard. This one I recognise and have desperately tried to ignore, to pretend it wasn't happening- but I have admitted now it's there and asked for help some weeks back. This resulted in an assessment on Wednesday (as I've asked for counselling) and I was diagnosed with severe depression, again.

For months I have struggled, you have maybe guessed through the poetry. I can't begin to explain to you how depression works, what it's like and how you feel. You can ONLY know this if you have been there. I could easily stop here and just say- that's it. I won't go any further. Bear with me. But my gut instinct has always been to be truthful.

Depression is cruel. It strips you of your logical self, your hope, your feelings, your desire for anything, even life. You can walk around and pretend you're Ok; put the face on that people want or need to see, but inside you are screaming. You can only do this for so long; then it eventually wears you down and the cracks begin to show. You begin to feel the need to shut down, switching off your lights one by one. Numbness begins to take over and the darkness becomes greater than the light. You haven't just found yourself back at the edge of the cliff- you stepped right over it without even thinking. Suddenly you find yourself dangling over the edge of an abyss with fingertips gripping like hell because only now do you realise- you need help.

Every piece of me feels broken. I look at the pieces all over the floor, but I don't recognise a single piece. How the hell do I put me back together? Yoga doesn't have the same effect; this body doesn't work the same. I can't use my crutch in the same way- I don't even know where to start. I feel like the last 7 years have been some huge joke played on me from my last bout with depression. Did it really happen? Was I once that strong, agile, young looking, fun, wise? The photos tell me it did but I don't in anyway recognise the person I see every day now. She is alien to me, there is nothing of her I know or understand. Even her eyes are dead.

The cancer patient, I got her; that was an image I understood. It was hard, it was hell at times, yes; but it was a battle I could see. And god forgive me, I have wished for her to return, because it's her I know. You see better people than you facing the battle still, and you wonder why them? How come it isn't me? They don't deserve it! They have too much to live for! And then you look back at yourself, the person who is slowly shutting down. Depression is invisible; you are fighting blindly because you don't even know who you are anymore.

I have asked for help and I am getting it. I have those closest to me, my incredible girls, Neo, my family and of course, I have my tribe still. I have been brutally truthful to you. If you choose to judge me, then that is your choice. I didn't ask for this, it came. As Wendy has said, look what came out of my other depression. So, do I know what's coming? No. I can only look to here and now. I am at 'Ground Zero'.

3rd December 2017

Yesterday I held up my hands and admitted that I was again suffering from depression. Is this cancer trying to have a last ditch attempt to kill me? My mind has been battling a while, the thoughts I have been having are so, so wrong. Yet they say this is completely normal, to question- 'Why am I still here?' 'Why are others still fighting and not me?' I have been diagnosed with severe depression, but it is a place I have been before and somehow survived. I would say to those who can't understand it- Depression is the Cancer of the mind.

I Am She

She hadn't seen it coming, though the warning signs were there.
Invisible, insidious, the 'Black Dog' stripped her bare.
The mountain she had climbed this year,
seemed gentle in it's wake.
What faced her now... like Everest, on this her soul could break.

She knew it all, the world of Google played within her hand.
'Feelings After Cancer' threads, to help her understand.
But nowhere did she seem to find,
the thoughts that plagued her head.
While others feared it might return... she felt a hope, not dread.

She saw the others round her fight, the battle she had won.
Amazing women, mothers, girls... just not the place for some.
And randomly it seemed to take, the ones who least deserved.
She couldn't see or understand, why she had not been served?

A bitter guilt engulfed her mind...
Why them? And why not her?
Their lives so precious, hers was not. Her logic was a blur.
Then memories and echoes cried, those words she'd heard before.
Oh God, she was again, in Hell. Depression had the floor.

How had she missed how close she was?
That cliff was bearing down.
Without a thought, she'd took that step.
So slowly she would drown.
And now she clung, with fingers gripped,
from depths that welcome call...
"Go on, let go, you know you must. Into the darkness fall."

It felt so easy, letting go. Just let depression win.
She'd fought this once,
she knew the drill... quell voices from within.
But where to start? Her yoga mat no longer held the key.
Instead, it now just made it worse, her body wasn't free.

118

For cancer and it's treatment had, left side effects so cruel.
No longer could she hold her pose, it's energy to fuel.
The very thing she knew would help, it left her feeling weak.
There had to be another way, allow her soul to speak.

She knew her tribe of warriors, around her they would fight.
If poses couldn't help her now, then maybe she could write?
Each time she felt that darkness come, her pen to paper place?
To call for help? This battle now, alone she couldn't face.

The pieces of her broken self, lay scattered all around.
But sifting through, not recognise a single piece she found.
The cancer patient, her she knew. That fight she understood.
No wonder that her wishes were... return to that she would.

For this was cancer's final knife. Content with body? No.
This evil bastard went for mind. To have it's final blow.
Somewhere within, she made that choice.
She knew she had to cope.
Herself, her girls, the ones she loved;
for them she would find hope.

Edwina Maria Thompson
© 2017

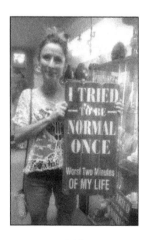

6th December 2017

It's A Wonderful Life

Has anyone ever seen this film? If you haven't, you really should. It has the most heart breaking but uplifting story line and moral to it. It never fails to bring me to tears by the end; in my opinion it's absolutely the best Christmas film ever made. It has James Stewart in it and it is possibly the performance of his career. Ironically, I learnt recently that he was suffering from PTSD when he was filming his scenes. No wonder his acting is so moving and powerful- his tears and pain were real.

You're probably wondering why I've brought this film up... it came to me today when I had to discuss my finances. (I decided I'd had enough of worrying about a loan I have from years ago and I'm letting Stepchange sort it out.) They were all fab and I am feeling a little better knowing that things are going to be dealt with.

Anyway, I digress again- the point I actually wanted to make was about money or lack of it. As you know I've been diagnosed with depression (counselling begins this week), so discussing such serious things wasn't easy. I had to relay what my monetary assets were and what I was actually worth. It was easy to answer- £200, the cost of my 25 year old car. No house, no savings, just a car. Then it struck me... was that all I was worth, 200 quid? My God, after 25 years of working and teaching, was that all I had to show for it? Then I remembered my teacher's pension. I had that but it obviously couldn't be touched yet and it was there for my girls if I didn't survive cancer.

It was then that it hit me, just as it does George in the film- I was worth more dead than alive. It's a hellish thought, to know you are worth more dead. I've seen the film enough times to know the lesson that must be learnt from this. I don't care how much I have, how much I'm worth, how much I can leave behind: I know that I am surrounded by love and kindness. I have amazing people that love me, beautiful daughters, my partner, my mum, friends, family, my tribe and Neo. This is worth more than all of the money in the world. A fact we too often forget. So maybe when my head is at its worst... I can remember I am worth more than anyone can count in coins. I am worth more than an old car and a pension I can't touch. Money means nothing and shows nothing of who we really are. Don't ever forget that! Just as George learns how precious his life is and how much his very existence has touched others and helped to shape their lives- so have I.

8th December 2017

I have given in with my hair and tomorrow, thank God, Hayley will be dying it. It has depressed me more and more the longer it has got and especially as the grey became more obvious. I was even told I look like a grandma on Monday by my daughter's boyfriend. Curly was one thing, but curly and grey was just too much. I am not quite the 'blue rinse and set' brigade yet. So I say goodbye to my grey and to my 'Peter Shilton' look. Thank you for that one Lynn, I did look him up and I do look like him you cheeky sod. It's a bloody good job that I love you!

THE FIRST PIECE

10th December 2017

I think I'm going to call this- 'The First Piece'. My 'Nana hair' as Julie calls it, has finally gone. 12 months to the day this picture was taken, and considering the year I've had, it shows hope. This is the first piece of my jigsaw, the beginning of putting another me back together again.

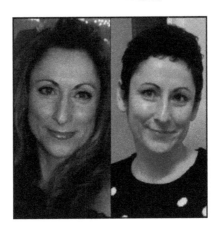

12th December 2017

Throughout my journey, I've gotten to know many amazing women from all over the world. I have had unbelievable support personally and have been lucky in this respect. However, one common denominator I have seen time and again- is that each of us seems to know that 'one person'. The person who you expected would help, but actually ran a mile as soon as you were diagnosed. The person who acted like they would 'catch' the cancer from you and avoided any contact with you at all times. You wouldn't think that anyone would be like that in this day and age, but they are. So for those ladies and men who have known someone like this… this one is for you.

<u>Where Were You?</u>

This journey took me places that I never thought I'd be.
I've made new friends, the best there is.
I've learnt who's there for me.
But still the question haunts my mind,
it never sets me free.
Where were you?

The one I love was by my side, as we faced 'no man's land'.
And through my hell, we've laughed,
we've cried; he's always held my hand.
Yet still the question won't die out,
it cannot understand...
Where were you?

When I was weak, he washed my hair,
and gently rubbed it dry.
When time it came to shave my head,
he kept my spirits high.
So here I find, I'm asking still.
I just want to know why...
Where were you?

My kids have been amazing, I'm so proud in every way.
I couldn't wish for anymore, my love it grows each day.
But there it is, that question still,
it will not go away...
Where were you?

The warriors and even strangers never let me down.
With coffee, cakes and thoughtful words,
they always were around.
So tell me why the question here,
forever makes me frown...
Where were you?

You never came to treatments or took time to visit here.
You never even tried to phone, and lend a friendly ear.
No longer will I waste my thoughts or shed a single tear...
Not for you.

Edwina Maria Thompson
© 2017

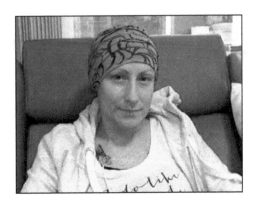

17th December 2017

This is a poem I have had great fun writing. It is a little bit in keeping with my previous poem, but this one goes even further. Not only are there people who go out of their way to ignore you, there are also those who go out of their way to hurt you! People who show absolutely no empathy, compassion or understanding of what you are going through. There is little you can do about people like that, you can only leave them in their egotistical ignorant worlds and walk away. This poem is for a wonderful TNBC warrior who is dealing with exactly that kind of person right now. I hope this makes her and a few out there giggle!

Some People

Some people are just shits,
No matter what you do.
They'll try to hide with rosy scent,
But shit will still seep through.

So visualize a box,
To put all your shits in.
Make sure that you have sealed it tight,
And throw it in the bin.

Then leave it there a while,
To fester and mature.
You never know, some time might turn,
Your shits into manure!

Edwina Maria Thompson
© 2017

24th December 2017

I've just been to Julie's to exchange pressies for Christmas. She's very impressed with herself; she's made a Christmas cake- from scratch! Not something I think I could do. She had to do the preparations for it months ago and I don't think I have the patience for all that. I do love Christmas, everyone's decorations always look fab and of course Michael Buble has to be on repeat for a month. Not to mention it's a great excuse to add a tiny bit of Baileys to my coffee every night! (My waist line and thighs might regret that come January though.) We even went to a Carol concert the other night; wrapped up in scarves, gloves and hats to keep warm. I've not been to a proper church Christmas Carol concert in many years, and I absolutely loved it. There's nothing like belting out 'Oh Come All Ye Faithful' surrounded by candlelight to remind you of how precious life truly is. Yep, It's A Wonderful Life.

25th December 2017

What a fab day I've had. I spent the whole day chilling out, (Christmas dinner with the girls is tomorrow.) Then listening to George Michael this morning, thinking to myself: how lucky I am to be here. I plan to watch another of my favourite films by tonight too: The Muppet Christmas Carol. You can't beat those songs on Christmas Day! Last year Christmas Day was a little uneasy as I was waiting for the results of my biopsy; but this year... I've come through it all. Yes, there's been cancer, treatments and depression but also friends and family, so I am still overwhelmingly happy. I simply couldn't ask for a better present, my health. So I say, a very Merry Christmas to one and all.

27th December 2017

One of the things that has really shocked me during this journey, has been the behaviour of a few people. I've been blessed throughout with support and have never had to cope alone; but I know of many who do. I've been told of partners, friends and family moaning about their colds, coughs and little niggles... to someone going through cancer. (Not me luckily I might add!) You do think to yourself, get a bloody grip... try this game instead. Now that would give them something to complain about! So, if you know of someone facing this battle, text them right now and just say 'How are you doing? I'm thinking of you.' Remember how lucky you are, not to be in their shoes.

Would You?

Would you walk in my shoes for one day?
Would you want to be cut open, poisoned and fried?
Would you dread all the treatments for months on this ride?
Would you thank God for those who had stayed by your side?
Would you walk in my shoes for one day?

Would you handle this journey alone?
Would you need someone there for results when you're told?
Would you go to your chemo with no hand to hold?
Would you struggle unaided the more you feel old?
Would you handle this journey alone?

Would you feel like it never will end?
Would you cry when you wake to find clumps of lost hair?
Would you cover your head so the people don't stare?
Would you recognise 'you' when your face becomes bare?
Would you feel like it never will end?

Would you carry that ticking bomb round?
Would you tackle the demons which torture your mind?
Would you welcome and suffer the pain each day finds?
Would you hope you could leave all your fears behind?
Would you carry that ticking bomb round?

Would you walk in my shoes for one day?
Would you have to seek help just in order to cope?
Would you conquer those demons and walk this tightrope?
Would face your new future and life with great hope?
Would you walk in my shoes for one day?

Edwina Maria Thompson
© 2017

28th December 2017

A New Year, A New Hope

Every year at Christmas in my yoga class, I tell a story called 'The Best Christmas Present in the World' by Michael Morpurgo. It is a story about the cease fire in no-man's land on Christmas Day 1914. That same event was depicted in the Christmas song 'Pipes of Peace' by Paul McCartney, which has popped up on TV a fair few times this week. The other day I watched Doctor Who and again, that event was dramatised. I've always been very moved by it, that for just one day, enemies came together and shared Christmas as one. Then today, I saw something on a programme which made that event even more moving and selfless than I had ever realised.

In the 1st World War, as the conflict spread, Britain's supply of sugar from the continent was greatly reduced, (up to 80%, as had happened to Tate in York.) Companies had to slash their products, and chocolate became even more precious than ever. Despite this, in Christmas of 1914, the Sheriff of York and the Mayor had thousands of boxes of chocolate sent to the boys on the front line. This was to boost their morale, receiving a little something from home. Many men wrote back, so touched by the gesture and so grateful; that they wanted to say thank you. In one letter, a young man said...

"I should like to have spent Christmas at home with my parents. But duty before pleasure. I am looking forward to a speedy termination of this cruel war. I shall prize the box of chocolates, as long as God spares me. One never knows what a day brings forth."

The young man whose words these are, Henry Bailey, died shortly after he wrote it. So many of them thought they would be home for Christmas, but as we know now, that war went on and killed hundreds of thousands.

What struck me was, here they were given something so precious, that they wrote home to say thank you. But if you know anything about the Christmas Day truce, one of the things the men shared, was chocolate. They were willing to share something so treasured, with their enemies. Even if just for one day, they had compassion, empathy and understanding for each other. Actually, it wasn't the only truce: there had been many outbreaks along the front line where the two sides had come together. So, as you can imagine, by the big Christmas Day truce, High Command had had enough and put a stop to it. Men were threatened with being shot for mutiny. They feared the men would question the war... and the men at the top couldn't have that.

Over a hundred years later, we can learn a lot from those young men. Whoever the first man to wave that white flag was, my god he must have had some balls and strong feelings of hope with a trust in humanity. We live in a world that is rich with beauty, purity, kindness and love. But also one that feeds us fear, jealousy, hatred, envy, greed, prejudice, anger, lies... I could go on. A world were social media allows two of the most power hungry men on the planet, to argue/name call on Twitter like schoolboys. A world of an elite that tries to control people with fear. So it does take a lot of strength and courage to stand up against those kind of people. However, if we all did it- can you imagine the world we would live in! Sometimes it only takes one or two... just look at Rose McGowan and how she empowered a tidal wave of women and men to speak out. #metoo

This year I've seen the best and the worst of people, sometimes from my own experiences and sometimes from those of others. I've seen kindness, love, great compassion and empathy. I've been lifted by so many of you throughout the year, it truly overwhelms me. I have had to change my own opinions and beliefs in many ways which has taught me one huge lesson...

you cannot judge a person's actions or beliefs until you walk in their shoes.

12 months ago, I knew nothing of cancer and genuinely believed chemotherapy was a huge con. Here I stand now, having taken that option because I am far better educated about the disease itself, than I was then. There are over 200 types of Cancer. Even within my own, Triple Negative, there are 6 subtypes, meaning that treatments don't always necessarily work the same. Treatments are often a shot in the dark. Thank God that so much money has been put to TN research; even in 12 months I've seen how much has been learnt and developed. Do I still believe we should be given access to cannabis as it heals many cancers? Yes I do. Would I take that option in the future if I needed to? Again, yes. However, I would also be willing to go down the conventional route again too. I have changed my beliefs, because I have now walked the path of Cancer. I walked in those shoes so now I understand.

I am so looking forward to 2018. I look to the New Year with an entirely different set of beliefs, hopes, gratitude and expectations. I'm learning never to underestimate myself, finding new ways to 'pay it forward' and discovering skills I never even knew I had. I will continue as best I can: to always see the goodness first and be ready to love, forgive, trust and hope. I have faith in humankind. Also, I like to think, had it been me on the front line all those years ago... I would have been one of the first to wave that white flag- and maybe I would have even shared my chocolate.

2nd January 2018

Happy New Year to you all! I have a New Year's resolution, one I have NEVER had before: to lose the extra weight. (Unfortunately I can't blame all of it on treatment side effects; some of it is massive over indulgence at Christmas like the daily Baileys!) I more or less have the aches and pains under control with medication now (I'm drugged up daily with Amitriptyline and Lyrica); and my mind is being sorted through counselling. I'm still being extra careful with poses, but today I just couldn't resist. I'm in a different house, with different hair, a different body, a 4 legged friend and a modified easier pose, but I'm still there. I am stronger, tougher, wiser, kinder and of course, forever the warrior. Break me as much as you can... but I will always be able to stand on my head. I have found my new wings yet again.

New Wings

There once was a time when my soul was a mess,
And suicide seemed the way out, I confess.
I searched round for answers and prayed for a sign.
From darkness, a light that would break through and shine.

The universe sent me an angel to guide,
She led me though yoga, and stayed at my side.
One pose that she taught me, it gave me such fight.
In headstand I gained, not just strength but insight.

My world upside down had a different view.
I saw I could conquer whatever life threw.
I'd roll up my mat with new power and force.
I vowed then, how nothing could break me, of course.

The universe smiled as it watched me come through.
It left me for years building my 'self' anew.
I had no idea though, that more was in-store.
A new set of wings, greater heights there to soar.

The challenge this time wasn't just heart and thought.
My body now damaged, with cancer it brought.
It gave to me battles that tortured my soul.
And left me to work out a new set of goals.

I've laughed and I've cried, but I've learnt through this war.
To never be broken or doubt what it's for.
These battles and challenges we have been thrown.
They're all there as lessons, each one is our own.

I look to the universe now this New Year,
I've come through your journey, my thanks are sincere.
You gave me once headstand, and all that it brings.
So now I'm again flying high... with new wings.

Edwina Maria Thompson
© 2018

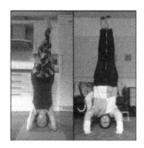

5th January 2018

A Year Has Passed

Tomorrow is January 6th, and to most of you that date will mean absolutely nothing. To me it's a year to the day I was diagnosed with cancer, my 'Cancerversary'.

I'll be honest with you, looking back very little of it actually feels real. The only things that remind me daily of what happened are my side effects and the mirror. I guess in the beginning I was probably in shock, even though I had known for a long time that something was very wrong. Ironic isn't it: at the point I felt my strongest and thought I looked my absolute best, I was in reality very ill. I had a disease that had the potential to kill me (and still does), but I had no idea.

This journey has taught me a lot. I have learnt to appreciate every single thing in my life: my children, my family and friends, my health and my job. I have probably learnt more about yoga and how it helps you to live your life... 'off my mat', more than I ever learnt 'on it'. You see, life really is far too short, whatever you believe in. You will live this life you have now, only once. Are you doing what makes you feel good; or at least what makes you content- maybe even happy? If not, then how can you change that? I wish I could wave a magic wand and give everybody their dreams, but I can't. I can only encourage you to achieve yours.

A year has passed and slowly but surely, I'm getting to know this new me. I prefer her. A lot of the good stuff from the old me is still there, but now with much more compassion, acceptance and patience. This one also says it as it is, she doesn't hold back! (I think her 'f**k off' button is broken to be honest.) I've made my goals for this year; one of them is to get back into a few of those poses on my medical booklet: 'I can and I will'. Just watch me.

One year, that's all it takes for huge change. Look at the changes I went through last year, they were pretty massive. Make that decision for tomorrow and begin to make the changes you want. Let January 6th be a special day for you too, the day you put your dreams in motion.

6th January 2018

Wow, a year to the day I was diagnosed and I am back learning on my mat. I am studying Yoga Nidra at a weekend workshop with the Yoga Nidra Network. Isn't it amazing how resilient the human spirit can be? Only 4 months ago I couldn't even face rolling out my mat, and now I'm here. I love this type of yoga so much, pure relaxation for the body and mind. You don't have to do a thing, no poses, just lie there and listen. My absolute heaven. Yoga of course, was always about my heart and soul, so this is perfect for me.

SO MANY JOURNEYS

9th January 2018

I've written this for my warrior friend Julie. It stems from a conversation we were having recently about the days she doesn't even want to get out of bed- days when everything just becomes too much. I was explaining to her how I tend to call those, "Hippo Days', when you just want to wallow and hide away. There are times we all have Hippo Days, and they truly help us to heal and make us appreciate all the tiny but wonderful things in life. Without them we would just carry the hurt around. I can't lay claim to the phrase 'Hippo Day' that came from another warrior friend, when I needed to know how important these down days are.

I write an edit to this as I place all of my work into this book. After Julie's tragic and untimely death from Triple Negative breast cancer, her family asked if there were any of my poems which could be read at her funeral. This was the poem which was chosen, and read by her brother David. As her family said, Julie would often refer to herself as having a 'Hippo Day'. I know it holds a special place in their hearts, as it does mine. For Julie.

<u>Hippo Days</u>

Today I need a Hippo Day,
To wallow, scream and cry.
If I don't have my Hippo Days,
I think inside I'd die.

My Hippo Days are there to heal,
They help release my pain.
I sink and drown in my own mud,
No sunshine there, just rain.

I scream about how wrong this is,
I'm fighting for my life!
While others sweat their little things,
They've no idea of strife.

It always breaks my heart to hear,
The problems we create.
Just why the world can't get along,
Without this fear and hate.

I really wish that everyone,
For one day could receive,
A chance to see life through my eyes.
For their old self, to grieve.

I'd let them have these Hippo Days,
And have to search for light.
I'd let them wallow in my mud,
And pray for days more bright.

I wonder if then, they would see,
The thing so clear to me.
That life is such a precious gift,
But holds no guarantee.

I need to wallow for today,
And cry my tears dry.
But then I'll find my fight again,
This life won't pass me by.

I'll smell the flowers, dance in rain!
I'll cherish every smile.
I'll give my thanks for days like these,
My hope, they last awhile...

And when again my Hippo Days,
Bring tears and hurt to feel.
I'll even give my thanks to them,
In those, my heart will heal.

Edwina Maria Thompson
© 2018

14th January 2018

In my life I have known of far too many people who have died, and tragically died at a young age. I've learnt over and again how fragile life can be. Now, having had breast cancer, I'm in another world of so much joy, support and happiness, but also of loss. At times it is devastating to know how many hearts are being broken by this disease. I struggle to see any good in so much loss; there isn't as far as I can see. I feel so angry sometimes, lost, desperate to do something to help- but I can't. All I can do is hope, pray and write.

Cancer is cruel and vicious in all the forms that it takes. Too many have lost their lives to this disease and too many are facing the ultimate fear that a metastatic diagnosis brings. This is for all of those beautiful angels who have gone before, we will always remember.

<u>Too Many</u>

I'm sitting here with pen in hand, unsure of how to start...
Too many women suffering, too many broken hearts.

Too many children lost in tears, another mother gone.
Too many partners left alone, when all is said and done.

Too many ladies fill my mind, supporting with their smiles.
The way each one had brought such love, to others over miles.

Too many families and friends, all shattered by their pain.
If only I could wave a wand... to make it right again.

Too many searching for some light, a way to guide us through.
Too many times we say goodbyes, to those we loved and knew.

All those lessons I have learnt, how life is but a blink.
A spark in Mother Nature's eye, just pause a while and think.

We need to balance out this pain, and bring some light and love.
In memory of angels passed, too many up above.

Immerse our lives with hope and hugs, so many kisses give.
So many times to pause and breathe, remembering to live.

So many moments, cherish now. Not one of us can know,
Quite when our time on earth will end, that last act in our show.

So many positives are there, you only have to look.
It's up to you to search and find, this life holds no handbook.

Please take this moment now to smile, light up your perfect face.
And promise those whose hearts we've lost,
we'll honour them with grace.

Edwina Maria Thompson
© 2018

16th January 2018

I went round to Julie's today for a catch up. She is struggling a lot recently, but just as much with her mind as physically. I gave her a mantra of me singing some months ago, which she absolutely loves to listen to. (Sanskrit words can have a very powerful effect on the body and mind.) So I've said we must go to a yoga class together and see if yoga can help her too. We chatted a lot about this disease, what an utter bastard it is. The loss of one of our warriors in the group has hit her hard. TN is so unpredictable… you just don't know what's going to happen. I have a few meditations I said I would send to her; I know they can't wave any magic wand, but maybe at least they could give her mind a respite. Yoga was able to pull me from depression all those years ago, so I desperately hope that it can help if just a little.

23rd Jan 2018

I've got a catch 22 and I can't make up my mind. The doctor has given me Naproxen and Ranitidine for my back (when it's bad my whole body is sedentary and painful, especially when I don't take the pills.) The problem is, the bloody pills make me constipated (this is the second lot of drugs he's trying me on because of that). If you have ever suffered from constipation, you will know what it is like: everything stops and you feel like shit! (Excuse the pun). So my dilemma is back pain or constipation, which do I choose? I've not taken any pills today in the hopes that I'll go! The consequence of that is that now my back is playing up again. Argh! I've tried 3 days of back pills with fibre drinks and Senokot to move things, (alongside yoga twists)… and bloody nothing. This whole thing is driving me nuts!

1st February 2018

Today I had a lovely get together with some of my old TN Warrior friends, Julie and Cath. It's wonderful that we all live so close, and now we have been joined by another warrior,

Joanne Binks! It's such a blessing to be able to meet ladies as they begin their journey, I think seeing some of us on the 'other side' of treatment must help a little. Now our hair is growing out though, we don't look as much of a 'club' anymore! Julie was struggling today though. Her body is reacting to the chemo and steroids now but she still had the biggest smile of us all. She truly amazes me.

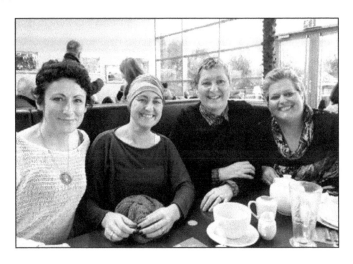

5th February 2018

Everything Changes

I've not been writing much recently because I've been very busy at home. (All will be revealed). I'm slowly getting back to classes but using some common sense and watching my back, (I am having some serious issues and problems with it.) It was amazing to get back into headstand though and I even attempted a handstand! My back didn't thank me for it; however, so I'm being sensible again. (I'm finally learning!) I am due to have an MRI to check the problems in my back aren't cancer related as well. Hopefully, once I've had my MRI and I know what's going on (all clear fingers crossed)... there will be no stopping me!

I believe it's thanks to so many that I'm here, fighting strong every day. My counselling is coming to an end shortly, and even my counsellor has been astounded at the way I was able to bounce back. Once I had recognised I was back in depression, I knew exactly how to get out! Teaching again at first, I found so difficult. I can hardly even remember teaching before Christmas, my mind was so screwed up and I was in a place of hell. Then two weeks ago, I came home and said to my girls, 'My God, I really enjoyed tonight!' It was the first time I had felt alive again teaching; I felt in control, content and at peace with it all. Everything has changed and that's ok. All new things to learn and accept, but thank God my love for teaching yoga didn't change; because for a good while there... I thought it had.

There's so much I want to do this year: - take on classes again, teach yoga in a gentler way, write a book, publish my poetry, do Reiki 2, see more of friends and my girls, appreciate the small things, lose weight, learn how to dance like they do on Strictly and take our dogs for long walks. (Yes, that was plural.) I've learnt that life is so short, and hugely unpredictable. I have no idea if I will be dead in 6 months (this is a reality I have to accept) or if I'll live to be a 95 year old, whippet loving, curly haired yogini, running a convalescence retreat with her aged partner in India. You just never know!

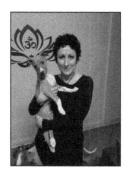

What I do know is, yes everything changes and that's all I can ever be sure of: but that's fine by me. I love my life and all of those who have brought such kindness, love, prayers, healing and compassion to me. If I died tomorrow I would be ready to go, because I already know I have lived a beautiful and full life.

So, with life being so short, I made another mad decision-meet the newest little addition to the madhouse, Sheru. He is our little lion (and Neo's half-brother). When Willow comes, (my daughter's' puppy) it really is crazy!

10th February 2018

I've noticed lots of people doing yoga recently, either getting back to it or trying it out as a beginner. I can't tell you how much yoga can help you. I'm an instructor myself of course, but I only found yoga at 40. Prior to that, I was desperately unfit and had absolutely no time for something as 'weird' as yoga! When I did try a class, I did it purely for my mind. It was a month after I had attempted suicide that I was dragged to a yoga class (Thank god.) From that moment on my life was turned around and only 10 months later, I was in India training as an instructor myself.

Yoga (if you find the right teacher and if you allow it) heals not only the body, but the soul. I highly recommend it. The physical benefits are just the bonus to be honest; they are the icing on the cake. For a while, I have been a little lost regards yoga (my passion alongside poetry): hence, I wrote the poem 'Drifting'. Slowly but surely as time passes, I am now regaining my strength and finding my way on my mat again. Be it through Yoga or through Poetry, I know I am meant to 'pay it forward'. My purpose is to help others like Callie, my beautiful yoga instructor and friend, did for me once. I'm also beginning to think that both yoga and poetry are very linked in my psyche, as I first began writing poetry when I went to India in 2011. Ironically, when I returned to India with my friend Angie in 2015 to study Yoga and Psychology; it was she who had always practised yoga not me... and I had thought of her as 'weird!'

So these two poems go back many years (one with a recent added ending). They are the first I ever wrote, 7 years ago in India.

For Callie, For Yoga, For Me

There was a time, not long ago,
When looking back was all I'd know.
My days were dark, my soul was black.
An evil clung onto my back.
I felt no hope, no will to live.
Alive, yet dead -nothing to give.
I begged each day, my pain would end.
But God a soul, he chose to send.

She made me cry, upon that floor,
But led me to an open door.
As months went by, I learnt to smile.
A thing I'd lost for such a while.
My angel spoke, each day I came,
My life to never be the same.

This angel left, my soul retained.
Yet in her place, a friend remained.
I thank you now, for so, so much.
And I've no doubt, you've more to touch.
For you can touch, the hearts you see.
But mine you saved, you gave me- me.

The years have passed, and I have grown.
So many lessons, I have known.
I've learnt to love, I've learnt to live.
And yet, I've so much more to give.

To pay it forward, just like you.
Be proud of me, I'm someone new.
And I still bless them every day,
To Callie, to Yoga, I found my way.

Edwina Maria Thompson
© 2011/7

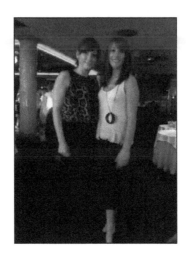

A Yogic Prayer

I roll my mat upon the floor,
The place, I find, where 'less is more'.
Through yoga I can live my Life,
Without the stress of daily strife.

A calming peace there lies in pose,
From tips of heads, right down to toes.
Breathing life to every pore,
Recharging on a yogic shore.

So let me thank, this time I take,
For every fall, I know I'll make.
You see, I know I'm truly blessed,
I gave my mind a chance to rest.

Namaste

Edwina Maria Thompson
© 2011

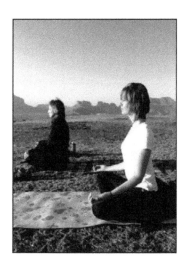

11th February 2018

This was me yesterday: a warrior to the core. Finally I'm getting back into the poses I love the most. Then from my determination arose another poem, yoga and poetry, so clearly conjoined in my head.

I actually had an MRI shortly after I attempted these poses and my god they're noisy! My back was pretty good yesterday (hence the Warriors with a few up dogs thrown in). Keeping on moving and strengthening my core, I know is the best thing I can do. So sod's law that lying static in an uncomfortable position for 40 minutes in a massive tunnel, set my back off again! The machine that's meant to tell me why it keeps becoming so painful- made it sore again. You have to laugh though I guess.

What I've come to realise, is that recovery is always three steps forward and two steps back, yes: but always still moving in the right direction... forwards and up! Tomorrow is my final counselling session and I have been blessed that I had such a wonderful person to help me: someone who got 'me'. So both my mind and my body are on the mend.

To be fair to myself, this is only a snapshot of how I am pro-gressing. I certainly couldn't keep these poses up for an hour; fifteen minutes and I'm done. Fitness wise, I'm definitely over halfway now but pain/numbness in my hands still causes many problems. (I might add, the radiographer said I wouldn't be back in a headstand for about 12 months but I said I'd do in in 6 months- and I did.) So do I have any words of wisdom? Not really, other than never doubt yourself! My mantra still: I can and I will.

Rise of the Warrior

I sense a burning from within, my soul ignites a flame.
The time has come for me to rise. 'Warriors' I reclaim.

Upon my mat, I find a peace, accepting what has passed.
That this is who I'm meant to be, I'm humbled to the last.

For all the angels we have lost, I dedicate to those.
Each gentle flowing movement made,
each precious breath, each pose.

With other warriors I faced, a challenge of great length.
Through treatments made to break us down,
From somewhere we found strength.

We've learnt to see the world through
eyes that cherish ev'rything.
As seasons pass, we just don't know,
Quite what the next will bring.

Warriors we have all become, to stand amongst the best.
I flow through poses now to show, how far we can progress.

My spirit soars, this heart, this mind. Warrior to the core.
This body moves with scars to tell, the battle it endured.

These poses ground me to the earth, then give me wings to fly
Advance, retreat, I bind, I bow. I raise my spirit high.

I thank each one for it's return, for never could I see.
Such fortitude would rise within, this yogi devotee.

For then I was a little lost, or maybe... I forgot,
That 'Yoga' is about the soul, just body, it is not.

The 'Warrior' reminds us that, ferocity exists.
But strength, integrity and love, we never should resist.

As Warrior, I am returned, all doubts and fears now gone.
Compassion, happiness preserved both off my mat and on.

Edwina Maria Thompson
© 2018

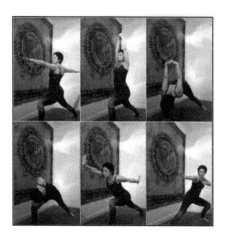

12th February 2018

Today I took Julie to her first Yin Yoga lesson at Lotusflower
yoga studio in Leigh. She has been having such a difficult time
recently; the visits to the hospital are never ending. She'll be
spending Valentine's Day having chemo again this year too.
I hoped that yoga and relaxation may help her a little, as it has
me on so many occasions and it did. She absolutely loved it! I
am so, so happy. In her own words, she felt relaxed. Fantastic!
I am so made up that we could do some yoga together. I better
get making my spare room into a yoga room, a little haven of
peace and calm. (And we were only a little disruptive in class,
I was very impressed.)

16ᵗʰ Feb 2018

Laxatives and Laughter

I've decided to share this little incident that happened to me last week. It was one of those scenarios where you think- this can only happen to me. I'll warn you, it's not pleasant!

I was going out for a few drinks with my friend Lynn, and I was dying to put on my new jeans (because they fit!) However, as I've been plagued with constipation since chemo, I decided to take Senokot, Fybrogel and Ducolose the day before our night out. This was to make sure 'I'd been'; otherwise those jeans wouldn't go on.

Of course Sod's law, 24 hours later- nothing. So I forced the jeans on and prayed the end result of copious amounts of laxatives would evade me. After a few hours of drinking, I felt it: in a packed pub. 'Bollocks' was my first thought, 'Oh my god, I'm going to have to go!' I left Lynn who was giggling away and legged it to the loo. Empty thank god! Anyway, said jeans decided coming off would be harder than getting on; but I eventually got them off and landed on the seat. I can only describe the next scenario in the words of Micky Flanagan the comedian- "With the gentlest of pushes, the world fell out of my arse!"

Not too bad you may think; but as this was happening a woman came in. I broke out into a panic. The noises along with the smell were horrific! So don't ask me why, but I thought catching it in tissue before it hit the water was a bright idea. It went everywhere on my hands! 'Oh my f***ing god, now what do I do?' Then just to top it off, I heard a scream of disgust along with a rant... "Oh Jesus Christ, what is that? Some people are disgusting! Who the hell would do that?!"....

'Oh bloody hell' I thought, 'I can't leave. I'm stuck here in my own shit, covered in it and drowning in my own smell. Now someone else is a witness!' I couldn't believe what was happening to me, it was like a bloody comedy show and I was the joke! I grabbed more tissues and desperately tried to clean myself up: in the process smearing shit just about everywhere on my backside. (Excuse the image!). After spitting on tissues and using my drink, I somehow managed to get myself clean.

Outside of my cubicle there was silence. I crept out and ran like hell for the sink to clean myself up properly. Hoping to God I got out before she emerged from her cubicle or anyone else entered. I desperately scrubbed my hands clean, but it was too late. Her loo door opened and I was caught... the culprit of the stench. She looked at me and said, "Oh my god, how disgusting is that!?" I raised my eyebrows, not sure how to respond. Then she pointed at the open loo next to mine. Somebody had vomited all over the floor, and there was poo all over the seat! "I only went and stood in it!" she cried. I looked down at the mess in disgust, "EW! Some people are absolute pigs aren't they," and then legged it right out of there!

Hee, hee, how lucky was I?!

20th February 2018

Woo Hoo! I have my MRI results back and there is no cancer in my spine, thank absolute God for that! It's been a real eye opener reading the problems picked up though. I have bulging discs, herniated discs, joint degeneration, degeneration in the pubic symphysis and tendinopathies. (Hmmm, no wonder my back hurts a lot). So I need to avoid forward bends, at least I know that. Yoga can certainly keep you fit but I think teaching the 17 classes a week I was doing, may have over done it with my body. Lesson learnt!

21st February 2018

A wonderful lady in my Triple Negative Warrior group recently had the worst news- that her cancer has spread. As soon as this happens to a fellow warrior, we are all devastated for them but we know that they will fight tooth and nail to beat this disease. We are often especially touched when it is someone who travelled the journey alongside us; someone diagnosed at a similar time.

I messaged Trine and asked if there was anything I could do for her, and there was. She asked me to write a poem for her, even giving me the title: "Three Weddings and A Funeral". Trine described what being given a 'secondaries' diagnosis is like in her own unique way... 'trying to hold onto diarrhoea'. I took her ideas, story and fabulous sense of humour; and wrote this. I was honoured that this poem was then read out by other warriors at her wedding. What an absolute pleasure and honour to write for you Trine, thank you! This is Trine's story.

Three Weddings and a Funeral

Three Weddings and a funeral,
(I know that should say Four),
But this one really is the last,
(I've not got time for more!)

You'd think that Dave had had his fill,
We fought this 2010.
But TN is the 'gift that gives',
So here we are... again.

We've been through shit, my kids and us,
Coz cancer strips you bare.
But on our Wedding Day, we win!
There's only love to share.

You have to laugh, or else you'd howl,
I'm just a 'tough old bird.'
Now 'secondaries'? I'm in the Club!
This whole thing seems absurd.

To hear the words, "You're now Stage Four"....
You're handed diarrhoea
Your life depends on holding tight.
Yeah right, what's NOT to fear?

You grab, but slowly watch it seep,
Through spaces in your hands.
Unless you've had to hold this shit,
You'll never understand.

But Cancer did forget one fact,
About his age old foe...
This Warrior does not stand down,
Her star sign is Virgo!

I'll sort my kids and post that Will,
My 'house in order' first.
Put ev'ry single thing in place,
Before he tries his worst!

My funeral, I might plan too!
Both dignified and fun.
I'll leave them laughing in the aisles,
And then my job is done.

For now, FUCK YOU! You think you've won?!
Dear Cancer, hear me say,
There's NOTHING that I will not try,
To fight you ev'ry way!

My daughters and my son will see,
This Warrior arise.
Even from the depths of Hell.
With fire in her eyes.

They'll see their mother grab each breath,
She doesn't plan to leave!
Like hell she'll miss her daughters grow,
Or ever make them grieve.

For Cancer causes death each day,
No advert can create.
The pain and heartache, tears and loss,
For me though, that WILL wait...

My name is Trine, I am more,
Than just this shit disease.
So love me now for all I am,
Let's laugh through life with ease.

Edwina Maria Thompson
© 2018

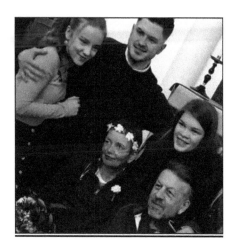

20th February 2018

I remember this day last year so well. I went into my oncologist's room on my own; I wanted no one with me. I took the decision at that moment I would take the route of chemotherapy. Up until then, I wasn't 100% sure. As a yoga instructor and very much into the 'alternative' style of treatments -I was strongly against chemotherapy. In my case it just seemed too much; but then I researched Triple Negative breast cancer and discovered what I was dealing with! I still believe there are some fantastic complimentary/alternative therapies out there, but I am also wholly aware that more aggressive forms of treatments are just as essential. If ever I am faced with a decision like that again, I will research and use my common sense first. I do however wish to see fairness across the board. ALL treatments, scans and genetic testing should be available to ALL patients, regardless of age, family history or postcode!

A Year Ago

A year ago today,
I signed my life away.
I chose to take 'chemo',
Although I didn't know.
Quite how it could change me,
Or help me better see.
That life is such a gift,
From which we shouldn't drift.
We need to see things clear,
Hold on to all that's dear.
To rise above the fog,
That clouds our minds like smog.
There's so much that we miss,
An ignorance of bliss.
So wrapped up in each day,
Too busy there to say.
We're lucky just to be,
A 'healthy, happy me.'
I know I'll not forget,
The special souls I've met.
Those friends who've brought me through,
And stuck to me like glue.
I send my thanks and praise,
My love and thoughts, always.
I'm humbled now to show,
How cancer helped me grow.
That life gave me this test,
For that, I'm truly blessed.

Edwina Maria Thompson
© 2018

22nd February 2018

Finally, the day has arrived. After many, many trips back and forth to the Christie hospital in Wigan and what feels like years of treatments- I have been signed off! I'll be honest; it felt at first a bit of an anti-climax. Then later on in the day, I went shopping and it hit me. There I was walking around Asda and I burst into tears for no reason whatsoever, other than it's all over and done. It feels like a huge weight has been lifted from my shoulders, but that another weight has replaced it. Somehow I have to find a 'new normal' from all of this now. I need to get to know this new me, find a way to work with this broken body and forge my new path in life. Thank god change never scares me and I'm always up for a challenge! Bring It On.

25th February 2018

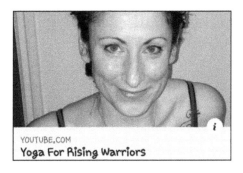

YOUTUBE.COM
Yoga For Rising Warriors

So, here I am! At long last I am beginning to put some yoga onto the Internet for anyone and everyone who wants to try some gentle yoga. I'll be posting videos of yoga poses, sequences, breathing (pranayama), meditations, yoga nidras (relaxations), chants and anything else that may be useful for well-being. I will target it for ladies/men who have come through breast cancer (or are still in treatments) but anyone can have a go to be honest. There is a Facebook group but also a YouTube channel, both of the same names. How excited am I?!

26th February 2018

When I wrote for Trine, I felt drawn to writing for my dear friend Julie on this day. Julie's cancer journey had taken so many cruel twists and turns, arriving in such an unpredictable and traumatic place, that I felt compelled to write for her too. I went back to the beginning of her journey, and told her story from when we first met. The last verses were added after she passed away and this beautiful picture was of Julie and Andy on Valentine's Day 2018. In her own words, "Love is... being with your wife while she has chemo on Valentine's day. #not-forthefirsttime." I truly hope there were angels who came to take her hands and guide her. Thank you to Julie's family for sharing her poem. This is Julie's Journey.

The Other Road

She had come to the end of her journey,
Along with some others she'd met.
Over months, they had all shared their stories;
Such empathy, soothed her mind set.

They would gather together for coffee.
(And stuffing their faces with grub).
Joking of side effects, warriors strong.
Soon looking like, part of a 'club'.

Hers though, had turned a more perilous path;
For chemo had not worked, at first.
Treatment had halted, mastectomy quick!
To lose her hair twice... she felt cursed.

But through chemo, they'd faced similar problems.
And talking, would help her off load.
Finally, each of her treatments were done,
A 'ring of the bell', now bestowed.

Still those niggles and worries, remained there.
She sensed that, it wasn't all done.
Thoughts in the back of her mind... were of fear.
It wasn't quite yet, a 'home run'.

Lumps then began, to appear on her skin;
But doctors, just fed her more pills.
Nobody, seemed to be anxious like her...
Coz instincts, were giving her chills.

She must shrug off those doubts, for her own sake.
The 'Future' to focus on now.
So, 'Moving Forward', she booked on the course;
With experts she might find out how?

Tears and laughter, were part of the day.
Some women felt just, as she did.
Part of her ready, to let go of dreads.
Find 'secondaries'... Heaven forbid.

Appointments 'following up', came around;
The radiotherapy last.
This time, the doctor seemed duly concerned...
Biopsies were taken, so fast.

Waiting felt endless, like holding her breath.
It just couldn't be, what she feared?
Please God, don't let any words be 'Stage Four'.
She prayed her unease, would be cleared.

Soon came the day, to find out all results.
As Andy held tight to her hand.
Nothing prepared her, for how she would feel.
Like free falling to, a crash land.

Words that had kept her, awake every night,
That voice, in her mind for so long.
"I'm sorry to tell you, yes, it has spread."
Her instincts were right... all along.

Everything deep in her belly, just sank.
Her world had been thrown, upside down.
Trying to listen, to plans put in place;
While slowly, she felt herself drown.

Chemo, again... but no loss of her hair?
Thank God, she escaped that old farce...
Trying to look on the funny side though;
'Breast cancer', was now on her arse!

Somewhere she found, there was courage within.
She'd fight all the way, in this war!
Anything now, she was ready to try.
With silver, oils, yoga and more.

This, 'other road', for the rest of her life?
Yes, 'cancer' was fiercely unjust.
'Terminal' though, not a word she would use!
But 'live for the moment', she must.

She'd face every day, the good and the bad.
Survivor! Her children would see.
Living her life, with the ones that she loved.
Despite cancer, she would be free!

And, now and again; her thoughts would drift to...
The angels, already gone by.
She'd light up a candle, drinking her wine.
Then raise, up to them, her glass high.

As months passed on by, angels gathered around.
Their hearts filled with sorrow and pain.
Yes time, it had come, for Julie to fly.
Such beautiful wings, would she gain.

Now watching above, like stars in the night.
Her love and her laughter, so near.
Deep in our hearts, her whisper is soft.
Hold memories of me... right here.

Edwina Maria Thompson
© 2018

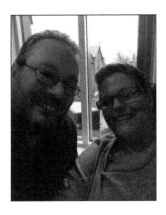

3rd March 2018
Triple Negative Awareness Day

Today is Triple Negative Awareness Day. All day I have thought about this and how I am (so far) unbelievably lucky. I want to share this blog from a wonderful young lady I know, Emma Knowles. If you have children who are young adults, ask them to read it. I'm being deadly serious here- you could save their lives. Make them check, make them know. This is the story of an amazing, strong, YOUNG and beautiful warrior- in her own words....

"Do you know what today is? Today is Triple Negative Breast Cancer Awareness Day. As someone diagnosed with triple negative breast cancer, I feel I'm in a good position to help educate a little bit today. After diagnosis, I researched a lot and I asked many, many questions. But it all seems to add up to a very dark picture. I'm told time and time again, triple negative has the highest death rates, it's the most 'complex' of cancers, it's incredibly aggressive, it doesn't respond to any hormonal treatment, there are higher recurrence risks.....I could go on and on and on. I've always liked to be 'special' but I can honestly stand here today and say omg I just wish I didn't have this rarer Breast cancer, I just wish mine wasn't so aggressive. But the facts are there in front of me. And my story alone is living proof of how traumatic a journey with triple negative breast cancer can be. I would never speak for others so I only tell my story....Triple Negative Breast cancer meant that many breast cancer treatments weren't available to me. So that cut the list of treatment down quickly. I've tried 5 different chemos and every time, my cancer has 'outwitted' it. I've had 5 operations to remove the bastard but still, it has always come back. I'm left hairless and full of scars. My arm has never been the same again. I've lain on machines quite literally frying my insides and I'm left with severe burns. My body has been PUMPED with drugs and at points I've even had to inject

162

myself. I've been in pain, I've been uncomfortable, I've nearly died, I've been brought back with the help of beautiful people who donate blood, I've lost mobility, I've lost my confidence, I've suffered financially and emotionally. All of this and I've only celebrated 28 birthdays. They say young women are more likely to get triple negative breast cancer and I'm sorry, but that SHOULD scare you! I always thought I was young, I was invincible, and those things do not happen to young women like me. But it did. And not only has it hit me hard but it's made my castle walls crumble and loved ones have had to rebuild me constantly. I carry guilt for my loved ones tears and the pain is torturous. Yet I've been the most open and honest with the world I've ever been. I feel a sense of responsibility to help you understand, to understand Triple negative breast cancer is no battle, it is a full on WAR. I've lost fellow warriors on the way and today I think of you. Today I also cry for the HUNDREDS of women I've connected with who also suffer the same diagnosis. I cry for their families too. Why!? Just why!? Why are there so many women DYING out there!? Why aren't we being taught about triple negative breast cancer? Why aren't these statistics being shoved in our faces? Why aren't we putting more money into specific targeted research? Why!? Why are the death rates so high!? Why!?

So, I ask just one small thing of you. I only ask that you take a measly two minutes of your day and Google Triple Negative Breast Cancer and just read something! Anything! Even just a few sentences! Look at the stats! Because trust me, they are quite horrifying to be honest.

I battle on in this war and I do it so well because of you! Long live Queen Bee."

THE TRUE WARRIOR

4th March 2018

Oh my god, what a start to the month. I am totally disgusted at a complete **** on the local retail car park, who's just forced me into oncoming traffic and nearly made me crash. When I got out of my car I saw red and went absolutely mental. He was sitting there in his big saloon car saying the same thing over and again, 'Learn how to drive your car'. So I told him, 'Driving a big flash car, you must be lacking in certain areas!' (I genuinely couldn't hold back. How dare he think he had the right of way just because he was driving a more expensive car?) I walked off in disgust but he wound down his window to shout after me- 'You know why people like you drive a shit car, because you haven't got a job!'

Well talk about a red flag to a bull! When I went back to tell him I drive a shit car because I've had cancer and had to return my newer one; he's bloody lucky I didn't punch him! He was actually shaking, gripping onto his steering wheel and hiding behind his rapidly wound up window. What a sad, cowardly and pathetic little man. He's probably never had anyone stand up to him so I hope that's taught him a lesson. He definitely wasn't expecting me to face up to him. It would seem that my fighting spirit is well and truly alive now. Hopefully that will teach him to show a little bit more respect on the roads, no matter how old someone's car is!

#cancerdidn'tbreakmeandneithercanyou

5th March 2018

The more I try and do on my yoga mat, the more problems I seem to be finding. I know that chemotherapy and radiotherapy leave side effects and problems behind, but I'll be honest- I didn't really think they would affect me in the way they have done. Waking up in the morning has become a bit of a farce; just trying to walk in a straight line is a challenge. I can't put my heels down from the pain, and my fingers are always frozen in a claw like grip. I spend a good 10 minutes every morning getting things working again- hands, feet, knees, back, neck and shoulders. I feel like I've aged 50 years over night without fail! What I am hoping, is that they will all eventually pass. The medication is definitely helping me, but I certainly don't want to be on that for the rest of my life. The doctor has already had to increase one of my pills to make it more effective, not something I had anticipated. I'm currently on triple the dosage of a pill my mother is on for arthritis, and she's 82! This has got to stop; I refuse to become reliant on pain killers. Then I remember though, I am lucky just to be here. I am alive and I am breathing, despite the 'Little Things'...

The Little Things

So here you are facing that new road ahead;
With hopes you can leave things behind...
But suddenly there are the after effects,
Taking over your body you find.

In the whole scheme of things, they really aren't much.
And you're thinking... at least I'm alive!
To look at you everyone thinks you're so well.
And expect that from now, you should thrive.

The problems you have, are the 'little things' left.
The 'gifts' that your treatments bestowed.
And most of these side effects, hidden from view...
In a body that's had overload.

You wake in the night from the fears and the thoughts.
That 'ticking bomb' loud in your dreams.
The worries and voices, that gnarl in your mind,
Just 'little things', really you deem.

As time passes by you, do put these aside;
And your mind becomes stronger each day.
Eventually you, 'find your feet', once again.
But in truth, you're not far from harm's way.

Those 'side effects' listed, were never a joke,
There's pain in my hands and my feet.
Sometimes it's tingling, but mainly they're sore.
And don't get me started on heat!

Hot flashes just come, with no warning signs there,
You're sweating, while outside there's ice!
Arthritis and joint pain now part of your life,
And as for your bowels... it's not nice!

Your hair, it grew back!! In most, rarely the same.
In all fairness, I do LOVE my curls.
My eyelashes though, they're so sparse, short and straight.
Mascara just can't make them twirl.

All 'Little Things', yes... but the list it goes on...
Neuropathy, menopause, creaks...
Restless legs, vertigo, scar tissue tight,
Your body is now an antique!

But actually I am the 'lucky one' here...
For now I can offer relief.
Through teaching and sharing, I'll reach just a few...
That 'Yoga' can help... my belief.

So here now I stand, facing life through new eyes,
I'll never forget what I've learnt.
And if I can soothe or relieve just one mind,
It was worth being poisoned and burnt.

Edwina Maria Thompson
© 2018

6th March 2018

I'm in the Leigh Observer this week, how amazing is that?
(I was a little anxious waiting to meet with the Reporter, just
in case he'd seen my rant on the Retail Park! It was all ok
though.) I'm so made up that this has got Triple Negative
Breast Cancer out there and it is as scary as it sounds. It was
Triple Negative Awareness Day on the 3rd March and we need
as much research, publicity and funding as we can get.

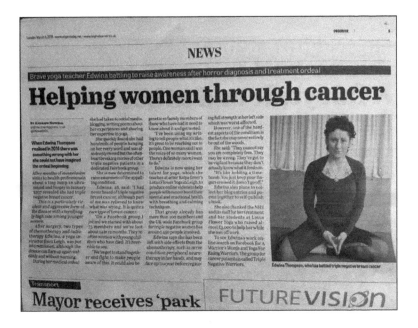

8th March 2018

I recently had an interview with Wigan Today about my journey through breast cancer. I am hoping that it will raise more awareness of Triple Negative breast cancer too. Hopefully one day, I can put my poems and blogs together into a book, and that may raise awareness too. It's been so strange watching myself on the news, even if it is only on the Internet. This disease is shit and we alone in my Triple Negative group have lost too many women. Too many have lost their fight and too many are now diagnosed with second-aries: each one a mother, wife, daughter, sister, aunty, niece or friend- all taken or broken by Triple Negative. TN is more common in younger women so I cannot urge you enough to check and know your body. If you are young yourself or know young women- let them be aware. Don't let them think they are too young to have breast cancer. Triple Negative needs to be known and shouted loud out there. There is no targeted treatment for TN and no pill to take after treatment to prevent it from returning. We are given yearly mammograms and that is it, despite statistics showing how evil and unpredictable this particular disease is. The NHS can only do so much for us, and then we are left to wait and hope.

13th March 2108

I have written so many poems about cancer, but never have I really thought of loss from a daughter's point of view. My thoughts always seem to be for a mother leaving her children, thinking from her point of view and how I would feel if I had to leave my children behind. My own mother is alive and well thank god, but I do know of too many people who have lost their mother or father to cancer. I think losing a parent is just as cruel and heart breaking, whatever age you are. (Losing anyone you love is heart-breaking of course.) So Dee, this one is for you and all of those who have lost a parent to this unforgiving disease.

She's Gone

I dream at night I see her face; a smile that lit the room.
A mother who had nurtured me,
each moment from her womb.
So many things I never said, the time it went too soon.
Now she's gone.

I think I hear her laugh sometimes, my memories so clear.
I close my eyes and smell her scent, it feels as if she's near.
Her spirit lingers comforting, within the atmosphere.
But she's gone.

I picture times we joked and talked,
both mother and my friend.
The thought just didn't cross my mind,
those chats would ever end.
The only person truly there,
on whom I could depend.
Yet, she's gone.

I watched her fight for every day,
as cancer sealed her fate.
I prayed, I begged,
God help her please... don't let it be too late.
But now I'm left with broken heart,
a burden of such weight.
Yes, she's gone.

Her whisper softens in my ear, "You really mustn't cry.
Remember me with hope and love, don't ever question why.
I'll never leave. I'm in your heart, that part of me can't die...
I'm right here."

Edwina Maria Thompson
© 2018

20th March 2018

Another lovely meet up today with Julie, Cath and Jo; (Bents must be making a fortune out of us.) It wasn't as light hearted today I'm afraid. Julie is really tired with it all, Joanne is beginning to struggle through her chemo now and Cath is preparing to go to a funeral of a friend who has died of cancer. This is the reality of our situations I guess, cancer is not exactly a party in the park is it? It is wonderful that we can all support and help each other though. I sat and stroked Julie's arm as she told us of her worst fears. She spoke of her husband Andy and the kids, Hannah and Sam; saying how proud she was of them all but how scared she was at the thought of leaving them behind without her. Julie was so kind to Jo despite her own heartbreak, helping to calm her fears of this bastard of a disease. She held Jo's hands and looked right into her eyes, telling her how- just because Julie's cancer had spread, didn't mean that Jo's would too. It was so important for Julie to tell Jo that. Unfortunately I had a message then off my partner, saying Sheru was poorly. Julie insisted I left to get him to the vets, as she said "Puppies can become very ill, very quickly." So I had to leave them early. A sad but a beautiful meet up. It felt very different today.

9th April 2018

Carpe Diem

I have been so ill on and off for the past few weeks, I feel like I've just taken 10 steps backwards. I am streaming with cold and a have dreadful rash at my biopsy site; but I am guessing it has come on from me simply doing too much. (Videos daily for my Yoga channel have floored me; when will I learn?) I have been ok one day, and in bed the next. So now I rest completely, I have to. My poor body can't take anymore.

This week has been an absolute hell on earth for some families. There have been too many deaths in a very short time from this bastard of a disease and I can't comprehend any of it. There are times when the world genuinely seems to be a place of pain, hurt, heartbreak, unfairness, cruelty, unkindness: the list could go on. I am trying to see it like Pandora's Box. No matter what horror comes or what life throws at you; somewhere beneath it all will lay hope. There has to be.

This all has made me think of the words "Carpe Diem". They were often said to me by my dad and I have truly tried to live by them. I can remember as a child, he used to say to me 'Seize the day Weenies, Carpe Diem'. (Yes that was my nickname I'm afraid). I think from a very young age, I probably did. I had a habit of wishing for things and they would just happen. I fancied the job of 'May Queen' at school- I was chosen. I wished I could go to Boarding School and the next thing is- my Head teacher is telling my parents there is an advert for a Scholarship to a school in Wales. I applied, did the exam- and got a place. It felt so simple in my eyes. I wanted to fall in love easily and get married- and I did. I wanted 2 children with only 15 months between them- and they arrived. Early on in my life, things just 'fell into my lap' for want of a better phrase. I literally did seize every opportunity that came my way.

I think, maybe for a while, I let that ability to seize an opportunity get out of hand. I got a little too wrapped up in the whirlwind of work, expectations, ego and 'having and wanting' more. I fell into the trap of thinking I had to compete with the world, be the best, have the best and expect the best! I let pride get in the way I believe, and we all know what they say about that. Now here I am, still seizing an opportunity when it comes my way but without the trappings of materialism. Even taking something bad, turning it around and making good of it. 'Carpe Diem' or 'seize the day', it is a great phrase to live by especially in light of recent tragedies I believe. So thank you Dad for that one.

Returning to here and now, I would say it's really my mother who has given me words to live by more recently. She has shown me that there is always hope, love and kindness out there. She has shown me how to live by her own love, compassion, empathy and non-judgement. Even in my darkest moments, she has reminded me daily of 'Carpe Diem' in her own way. So I thank her above everyone else. I chose love, kindness and hope every time. Even in the most horrific of circumstances, just like in Pandora's Box: hope will always come through.

23rd April 2018

I've just returned to the doctors over the rash I have by my biopsy scar, as it just seems to be getting worse. At first she said shingles because it's on one side, then she decided it wasn't and hasn't got a clue what it is. Brilliant! She actually sat there saying, 'What to do, what to do?' Something would be a good idea? It's not painful because everything is still numb, but it's really uncomfortable. She's given me an antibiotic and steroid cream to see if that helps. The worry never ever goes away. I can hear that 'tick, tick, tick' in my bloody head again.

1st May 2018

Just Julie and I at the garden centre today, Wyvale this time and it was a quiet one. We still managed to put the world to rights, but our conversations feel considerably more serious now. Despite this, Julie still managed to have me in fits of laughter; I don't think that false boob will ever sit still! They are trying a different chemotherapy again now, but she has ended up in hospital a few times with bloods too low to take the chemo. She can see herself when the treatment is working, as the lumps on her arm shrink a little. They kind of develop this 'halo' around them as they go down. So I am praying that this treatment works. I wish to god there was more they knew about TN, then the treatment would be more effective. It just feels like they have a tick list of options to go through, and little else. There are so many trials out there too, and you just presume you will be able to join one- but that isn't the case either. You have to pass a whole load of criteria to get onto the newest trials. So of course, not everyone gets that chance. The unfairness of the whole process is beyond me.

I brought some Kundalini yoga chants with me today though. It's definitely a more unusual kind of yoga, but I know Julie is up for trying anything! I put them onto a pen drive for her to download. I did feel like a bit of an idiot sitting there in the garden centre though, singing mantras while I demonstrated hand positions. (Mudras) I know how calming mantras can be and Julie already has a recording of me singing a mantra that she enjoys listening to. So maybe these will help a little. I might add, we didn't get any free drinks this time... we must not have looked thirsty enough!

17th May 2018

I've been very worried about Julie recently, so I decided to just turn up on the doorstep. When she doesn't answer my messages, I know it's not good! Andy took me upstairs to see her as she's been in bed for days, not at all well. (I knew something was wrong.) The pain is so much for her now she can hardly stand up. When I got upstairs, she was naked so she was rather embarrassed! I wasn't bothered, I was just incredibly glad to see her. It was awful to see how poorly this bastard is making her; I was shocked at how ill my friend is. She has lost so much weight and is struggling to eat at the moment. She's been living on cream crackers and butter as it's all she can keep down. Andy and the kids are doing their best to help her and doctors have been round, but nothing seems to be helping. Hopefully her appetite will improve and she will pick up a little. I know her family are all truly worried about her.

19th May 2018

We had another get together today at Bents. Julie had actually organised this one, but she was too poorly to go. It was lovely, but just not the same without her. We got to meet another lovely warrior though, Louise Brad! On my way home, I had a message from Julie's mum Shirley; they are all so desperately worried and she wanted to know if I had spoken to Julie recently. I was glad I could say I had seen her, but it prompted me to go again. So I messaged Julie, and thank god she was a lot more upbeat! She told me she was up and about, and even fancied some fish finger butties. That's all I needed to hear.

I raced round to the local shop to get anything I could to tempt her with. There were fish fingers but they were 2 days out of date. 'I'll let you have them half price' the owner said. 'No thanks' I thought, I'm not bloody giving Julie out of date food!' So I grabbed some Mars ice-creams, fish fingers and flap jacks and raced round. (I stopped at another shop for the fish fingers though.) It was fab seeing Julie looking much happier and brighter. She told me how she'd fell asleep in her chair the other day and hadn't heard her dad knocking on the front door. Next thing she woke up to him staring her right in the face and she nearly jumped out of her skin! I don't know who had the bigger fright! You gotta laugh though. So lovely that she's happier again now and she definitely looks a lot better. I know I call myself a warrior, but in all honestly -Julie is the true warrior here. No one has fight, bravery and strength like she does. As usual, the Tassimo went on and we sat chatting about life.

22nd May 2018

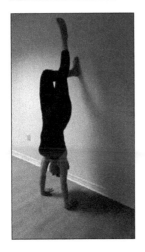

Sometimes when you look back, it's so hard to remember what you've been through. It seems now like a million years ago that I had no hair, eyebrows, strength or will even. You literally just get through by taking one day at a time. I might well be drugged up every day on pain killers and medication to help the side effects from chemo but I'm here and I'm alive. I've no idea what's around the corner, and so I take one step at a time. Breast surgery, chemotherapy, radiotherapy are all things that destroy not just the cancer, but so many parts of the body too. But today here I am- back in a handstand (if only briefly) and a massive thank you to Katya for getting me here!

23rd May 2018

They've kept Julie in again and aren't giving her the chemo. She was only doing the housework yesterday; she was feeling so much more positive about it all. She is not happy and posted a picture of her feet sat on the hospital bed. She hates being holed up inside. Hopefully this is just another blip.

25th May 2018

They are sending Julie for scans today. I have messaged her mum, and Shirley has said that Julie has deteriorated rapidly and is very, very poorly. I just don't understand what is happening, she was picking up. I've not told Cath though as she goes on holiday to Dubai soon and has had a lot on her plate recently. I am hoping that she doesn't need to know as yet. I am just praying with every breath I have now.

26th May 2018

Oh god, I have spoken to Julie's mum. It is the worst news, her cancer has spread more. They are saying she has weeks or months to live. This is a nightmare unfolding. I have phoned a few people in the group who are close to Julie and they are devastated.

27th May 2018

Shirley has messaged me and said I can visit Julie today. They don't think she is going to last the night. Everything has become numb.

SUNFLOWERS
AND PINK NAILS

28th May 2018

Julie Dawn Ainsworth sadly passed away from Triple Negative Breast Cancer on 28th May 2018. My love and prayers go always to her family and her friends. She is a lady who will be so deeply and sadly missed.

Today has been one of the most heart-breaking of my life. I was unable to sleep last night knowing how ill Julie was, and lay awake until 2am praying for that miracle to happen. I woke again at 5.30am and immediately messaged Julie's mum. Shirley replied, 'Our beautiful, loving and brave daughter lost her battle with the bastard at 12.58am'.

I am truly shocked by the loss of my friend and warrior sister. That this disease has chosen to take her is beyond my worst nightmares; I pray that wherever she is now, she is at peace and no longer in pain.

All day I have been receiving many wonderful messages of love, prayers and hope for Julie from our fellow warriors; everyone completely in shock as she was taken so ill, so quickly. Yet I knew that it was too late- Julie had already passed away in the night. When the time was right, all of the warriors were told the news and I have passed on the kind messages and prayers to Julie's family. I thank each and every one of these ladies for their love, support and kindness.

There is so much I could say about Julie, her kindness, love and compassion shone through her like a bright sun eradicating any shadow. Even within our Warrior group, she was forever thinking about how others felt and putting their feelings before her own. I am devastated to lose a friend so quickly, and heartbroken for her family. They were all with her at the end, and that is a blessing to know.

Julie's mother Shirley was kind enough to invite me to visit Julie whilst she was in hospital yesterday. I sat and held her hands, stroked her hair, talked about anything and everything and hoped in some way that she knew we were all there for her. Her brother, sister in law and nephew were with her too, so I asked her brother David if I could sing the mantra I had given her. He simply said, 'We will try anything now.' So I began to sing as I held Julie's hands and prayed that somehow this would help. I could only hope it eased her pain a little. I left when Andy, Hannah and Sam arrived. I thank them all dearly that I was able to kiss my friend goodbye.

As I drove home from the hospital, I could hear Julie's words in my head from our conversations, "I'm so scared Edwina." Everything felt like a surreal world evolving around me, where my brave friend was fading away. It was beyond anything I could ever have imagined. My mind was racing with what to do. I had asked for prayers to be said by the warriors just before I left the hospital, but I knew I had to let Cath know too and quickly. She was our other warrior friend, the third amigo. So I stopped the car to message her. It was the last thing I wanted to do as she was on holiday; finally escaping all of this hell. There was no easy way to tell her that Julie was so ill. We had both experienced too often what the outcome of this bastard could be. All we had left now was to pray for a miracle.

Today, with the sad news that Julie passed away in the night: I have chosen a sunflower to represent her. I feel that this shows what a shining light she was and always will be. She will forever hold a special place in our hearts.

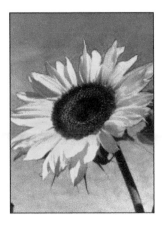

29th May 2018

Something incredible happened to me this morning. I received a gift that truly deserves a song of pure gratitude and bliss. No matter how heavy my heart is today; no matter how many times I've felt ill, hopeless or scared on this long journey; no matter how many times I looked in the mirror and didn't recognise the hollow person staring back at me; no matter how many tears I have shed for the many beautiful women we lost- this incredible gift still came to me every day.

This morning, I was given the gift of life- I woke up. And that is a gift I will continue to treasure, no matter what comes. So to all of those ladies no longer blessed with that gift and especially to my precious friend Julie; I will continue to treasure each day that I get to wake up

1st June 2018

This evening, I went to Julie's mum and dad. It was wonderful to be with her family, her mum Shirley, dad Colin, Andy,

Hannah and Sam were there too. We chatted about lots of things, Julie, her life, this disease, stories about the kids, so much. I laughed a lot; she certainly was a lady who leaves behind a huge amount of love. Her mum has been so overwhelmed to know how much Julie was loved and treasured, not just from the Triple Negative Warrior UK group too. She truly was a special soul. We chatted about how this disease feels like a lottery with no hard and fast rules. None of us really knows what will happen, as her dad calls it- a 'lucky dip'. Julie would want us to embrace life, even the Hippo Days; live every moment, grab it by the balls and fight every inch.

I thought as I was driving home, if it's a lottery then maybe we should turn it around. Rather than thinking we lose when things go wrong, let's see it that every day when we wake- we get to win the lottery. How blessed are we to have that, to see our lives as such a gift? May I never ever forget how lucky I am to be here.

2nd June 2018

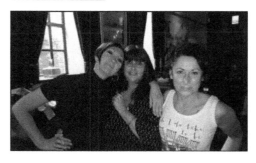

It has been lovely to get out with some old friends of mine, Angie Taylor and Lis Hughes who I have known for nearly 25 years. I truly wasn't in the mood for going out at all, but I think it did me good. We first met at a mother and baby group on 14th December 1994, and between us we have seen so much of life. I think it was exactly what I needed, a little normality. Although to call any of us normal is frankly pushing it. Love you both, my two utterly mad friends.

3rd June 2018

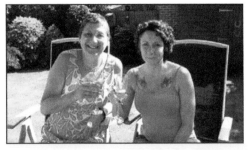

Cath is back from Dubai, thank god! I have been desperate to see her and to be able to talk to her about everything. I just needed to see somebody who 'got it'. I stopped off at the shops to get us a bottle of wine, and saw a pink one. It felt very fitting to raise some pink fizz to Julie's memory. We chatted about this whole shit disease and about the many times the three of us were together. It feels like a hole has appeared between the two of us. We are no longer complete, no longer the Three Amigos. We raised a glass high to our friend, she may not be with us in body- but she will remain a part of us in spirit as long as we both shall live.

5th June 2018

I have begun a little preparation for saying goodbye to Julie tomorrow. In keeping with her wishes and spirit, everyone will be wearing pink (many of us are painting our nails pink too): just as hers were in her last hours. I think it is a fitting and beautiful gesture to Julie, putting some colour and light into an otherwise heart breaking time. Thank you for that Julie.

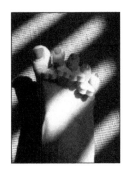

6th June 2018

Today was just a normal day for most. Not many people will have noticed how the whole world changed on 28th May 2018. There was an earthquake for me and so many people I have grown to love, but especially for one family- for them, their universe crumbled. Their beautiful Julie passed away. Today, we laid that incredible lady to rest.

This morning, Cath arrived at my house early; dressed head to toe in pink. She was a bag of nerves worried that she had overdone it with the pink; but just wanting to do something for Julie. It was such a lovely sunny day, I think pink was the perfect colour for us all. We got into Cath's car and left for the Crematorium, knowing we would be there far too early but neither of us knowing how to be or even what to say. None of it felt real, that Julie was gone. We spoke in the car of this evil bastard. We had known at the beginning that the chances were one of us would die, but never did we truly understand or believe that this was a reality. Never in our worst nightmares did we imagine it could happen so quickly.

When we arrived, friends and family were beginning to gather so we joined them outside. Cath though, was practically dancing about with needing the toilet and disappeared off. (She always needs a wee when she's nervous!) Of course, in perfect timing- I saw the cars begin to appear. I panicked and began knocking on the toilet door, urging Cath to hurry up. All the while thinking to myself, Bloody hell Julie- I can't take her any-where! (As I said to Cath later- it can only happen to you.) She got out just in the nick of time though and managed to rush to my side without getting herself knocked over....

We stood, side by side, the two amigos; as our dear warrior friend arrived in a beautiful hearse. Her coffin covered in her favourite yellow roses, with sunflowers interspersed to represent her fellow warriors. I was moved by how elegant Julie's daughter Hannah looked in her pale pink dress, so like her mum; and how smart both her husband Andy and son Sam were. I could just imagine Julie smiling down proudly at her precious family. Hannah stood with Cath and I while she waited for her grandparents and boyfriend to arrive in the other car. Cath later said, it was such a privilege for us to be able to stand with Hannah for those moments supporting her, as her mum would have wished us to do. We were soon joined by another of our warrior friends, Beverley-Anne and her friend and we all entered together.

Julie's funeral was beautiful. The room was full of course, so many had gathered together to say goodbye to such a wonderful lady. The ceremony was led by her cousin Chris and the words spoken about her couldn't have been more inspiring, touching and poignant. The songs were just perfect too. We laughed and we cried, and my spirit was lifted to hear the stories of Julie's life. Her brother David stood to read a poem I had written for Julie, 'Hippo Days'. He explained how Julie had often used this phrase, and how each of them now had many 'Hippo Days' ahead of them still. He read with poise and emotion, showing bravery that Julie would have been so proud of. I sat listening, arm in arm with Cath and Beverley-Anne; heartbroken but honoured to know my words had been chosen as a reading for her funeral. There was something so special to be there with Beverley-Anne and Cath. The three of us united in grief, in our rare cancer but in life too. Somehow I felt great strength in the three of us coming together for Julie, it is a feeling I shall never forget.

After the funeral, we all returned to Shirley and Colin's house. It was lovey to chat to so many and share our memories with her family. I had the chance to speak to David in the kitchen about the last time I had seen him and his sister in the hospital.

He told me how my singing had been a blessing for them. Julie had been agitated before I arrived at the hospital, but when I had begun to sing- the sounds seemed to calm and ease her: almost as if a weight had been lifted from her shoulders. I truly hope that in some way, those ancient words were able to sooth her path. I was also struck by how precious everything I had ever experienced must have been; that it had allowed me to do that for Julie in her last hours. The universe again weaving it's intricate web.

Today, three warriors stood united in grief for one whom we had loved and lost; but also united in hope that one day a cure may be found for this killer. I can't begin to explain how it feels to lose someone you love; to a disease that can take you just as easily and quickly. Cath herself was waiting for results of a scan after the wake today and this is the life we have to live. We have to learn to cherish every moment, just simply be grateful that we are still here- living each beauti- ful day. Julie's death came far too quickly and it has rocked the world of so, so many: her husband, children, brother, parents, family and friends. Today we said goodbye yes, but we celebrate your life Julie and promise that you will never, ever be forgotten.

9th June 2018

I've just rolled out Julie's yoga mat and bolster she bought to do yoga with me. Andy gave me all of the yoga things she'd bought, but was too poorly to do it. I've not been able to go into my yoga room since they were placed in there, the space I'd created for her and me to practice. But I realised they were bought to be used. Now each time I use them, she'll always be in my heart. Maybe one day I'll write a poem about her mat...

10th June 2018

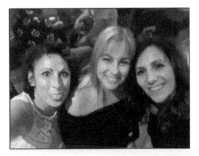

It was so lovely to get out again last night. It was the first time in a long, long time I've felt like I look 'normal' again. (Looking back at pictures from last June, it's been a journey to say the least, one that I'm still on of course.) Thank you Lynn and Carol for giving me a good laugh. The last few weeks have been heart breaking, but you gave me a well needed and massive lift. It was very much appreciated.

12th June 2018

Today Cath and I went back to Wyvale Garden Centre, the first place we all met up last year. The place where we had enjoyed free drinks because we talked so much! It was hard being there without Julie, I can't count the amount of times we visited there. It became like a second home to us for many months. We had to sit in a different place and not at 'our' table as they were cleaning; it just felt so different and empty. We sat and talked about Julie, sharing memories of our conversations. Cath said we had to move forward and take our memories with us. She is right. Julie would want us to live, enjoy life and absolutely make the most of it. Neither of us knows what the future holds, whether this time next year one of us will have gone too. We have to hold her memories close in our hearts, never forgetting what she means to us and to live our lives well.

14th June 2018

My heart seems to be entirely all over the place recently, like I'm waiting for floodgates to open. But nothing comes, only numbness. Even watching Love Island just brings smiles, rather than laughter. (Last year it got me through chemotherapy.) The only way I seem to be able to express myself, is through writing. So today I wrote again for Julie, of our last time together- adding to so many poems that I have written for her. I miss my warrior friend, as so many do.

My beautiful friend, warrior and angel, thank you for our many cherished moments. Thank you for inspiring so, so many of these poems. Thank you for being my rock in darker times. Thank you for the wise words and the laughter. Thank you for simply being you.

A Warrior's Goodbye

All I could do was hold your hands.
I had no magic wand.
I held the love of warriors,
I prayed you felt that bond.

I spoke to you, in hopes you heard,
Chatting of silly things.
Puppies, hair loss, coffee and nails.
Some comfort might it bring.

I stroked your hair, I held your gaze.
I hoped your pain would ease.
Unspoken prayers played on our lips,
Dear God, don't take her, please...

Our helplessness was all too real,
Yet watching, like a dream.
Your fears and instincts... coming true,
Your nightmare, now it seemed.

Haunted faces, dread in their eyes,
Their precious loved one lost?
Warrior sister and my friend,
We knew what cancer cost.

Remembered conversations, those
Of life and death we'd shared.
Inside my mind, your voice so clear...
"Edwina, I'm so scared..."

The heartache hanging in the air...
And nothing we could do.
Mantra now, was all I could give.
Yes, I would sing to you.

Gently holding your hands in mine,
I let the sounds begin.
A silence fell on all around,
Some peace might be within.

Powerful words from ages past,
Your favourite one, I knew.
Soothing, calming, song of my heart.
A prayer to guide you through.

I sensed your final hours had come,
And sang with broken heart.
Nothing, ever can prepare,
To see a soul depart.

Vibrations lingered in the room,
My only gift to leave.
I left as family entered in,
All hopes now felt naive.

Warrior sister, and my friend.
I got to say goodbye.
Go join the angels up above,
It's time for you to fly.

Edwina Maria Thompson
© 2018

18th June 2018

Wise Words

This is from a conversation with my very close friend last night, Wendy. She speaks volumes of cancer and it's fears; and she has experienced multiple tragedies from cancer in her own family. So she truly knows.

Me: I think it's just that it's not going. I'm numb 90% of the time. I desperately want to cry, scream and get it all out- but it's not happening. My body is slowly becoming tenser because I can't let go. I still can't believe what has happened. Part of it scares the absolute fucking shit out of me that it could be me just as easily; but I know I just have to accept that. I'm thinking Reiki is the answer to getting the tension out?

Wendy: Maybe it is. Maybe it's not. That's the thing with grief isn't it? It's different from one day to the next. Angry then bereft. The idea that it could be you any minute contradicts your 'first 5 years' laissez faire attitude of Que-Sera-sera- the yogic 'stay in the present moment' to the 'what if' of looking into the future. Don't force stuff, don't dwell too much. When it's ready it will all come out and if not- a coffee enema could always come in handy again!

Be kind to yourself though. I get the impression you don't know what to let out first. I'm wondering whether you need to sit and meditate a bit more rather than do yoga more. Try to feel what you're feeling at the moment in time with ahimsa (non-violence to yourself) and see how it changes/ shapes itself. It will come out when it's ready. I think it will come out when you understand what it is.

Cancer is so much more than a tumour. Even when the cells have gone, it's imprint is left forever. It's not about beating it

sometimes or winning some battle over it- it's about acknowl-
edging the damage it does and the power it has. Eventually,
like fighting the dementors in Harry Potter, you will build a
patronus. But sometimes it's the reality of knowing it can
really suck out your soul and there's nothing you can do about
it- even though you're fighting with your life.

Cancer shouldn't be underestimated in any shape or form. It's
so hard to say it needs respect but in a sick bastard kind of
way, in my experience- it does. I've acknowledged the damage
it can do in its greatest form. I celebrate the closeness, the love,
the fighting spirit & the relief it brings too. Like a dark
shadow- sometimes it leaves light. Sometimes it's nothing but
darkness and sorrow. Feel what you feel- when you feel it.
Don't force it. Be gentle. Letting go is hard to do when you feel
you'll be washed away by the flood.

Me: Thank you, as always you are making sense of the shit.
I am aware that it will hurt like hell when it goes: the last
time I finally let go of grief I had migraines for 2 days. Of
course, then I discovered my lump, so maybe it's fear that is
holding me back too. It breaks my heart that Julie didn't even
get 18 months, it is unbelievable. I have just got to 'go with
the flow' for the moment. Meditating is a bloody good idea
though, my brain is so like shit now I can't think of anything
practical.

Wendy: Some people don't get 18 weeks. That's one of the cru-
elest things about cancer. How does it decide who survives and
who passes within 6 weeks of a diagnosis? There's no way of
knowing. There's no way of trying to change it, it would seem.
That's why our feelings about it/ towards it change too: anger
that it's not fair; guilt that it's not you; fear that it could be;
despair at the hole left in the family and then hope that some
good will come of it somewhere, somehow. You said that to
me when we suffered with so much loss in our family. Be kind.

18th June 2018

It's strange how things happen in my little world. My mental and emotional health has been up and down like a yoyo recently. Yet this is good. Now I find this poem on my phone and I had no idea it was even there. I vaguely remember beginning it, but certainly not actually finishing it. At the time I was desperate to let all the hurt I had experienced go, but it just sat there leaving me numb and hollow within. I knew crying was the release I needed, but nothing came. So I wrote- and this was what I wrote, 'Let It Go'. Of course, these highs and lows are good; they are finally allowing me to begin a healing process. They are exactly what is needed right now.

Let It Go

Let it go people said,
Like I choose to hold on...
Numbing days, follow hours,
All the happiness gone.

Let it go, but where to?
Are they places to leave?
Do I box it all up?
With some calm to receive?

Let it go... yes, I know,
Rip it right from my heart.
Give me nights when I sleep,
Not a falling apart.

Let it go, sadness gone.
I can't bear much more weight.
Help me regain that hope,
No predicting my fate.

Let it go, find me light.
Give me highs and the lows.
Take the empty and numb,
Let me rest and repose.

Let it go, it's no good!
I can't hold all this hurt.
Let this spirit be free,
No more mind on alert.

Let it go, it is time.
Put the past all away.
No more looking too far,
Focus just on each day.

Let it go, but be kind.
Treat yourself with more care.
You will rise from the depths,
And your heart will repair.

Let them go, no more doubts,
Thank those angels who've passed.
Let them watch from above,
Find your peace at long last.

Edwina Maria Thompson
© 2018

22nd June 2018

So much has happened in these last few months. It's been an emotional rollercoaster. Things have happened which I've written about yes, but in no way ready to share. You get to the end of your journey, months pass by from end of treatment and people expect to see you back to your old self. It happened last year right so surely you should be over it by now? But you are never the same, you cannot be. You have experienced a world like no other and to not learn from that- not be more compassionate, not be more grateful for your health and life, not gain more humanity? Then that lesson, no matter how hellish it was, was a waste of your time and fight. But all of that to others, who don't know or understand, is very difficult to comprehend.

This poem is for the many warriors out there facing the trauma left by cancer every day. It is for those who are simply finding a way to be and act normal, when actually they often want to just run away and cry.

<u>Carry On</u>

So carry on regardless right...
That old 'stiff upper lip'.
Pretend it's dusted up and done.
Drop cancer 'membership'.

Just leave the groups who've got you through,
Forget the friends you've made.
It's not like cancer stays with you,
Best rip off that band aid.

So close your eyes, cover your ears,
Don't let more 'cancer' in.
It's easy just to 'let it go',
That 'new life' to begin.

Ignore the fears and doubts you have,
It's not like you'll be next.
Put on that fake smile every day,
Don't speak of side effects.

Remember you survived this shit,
They think that you're ok.
It's better not to let them know...
You want to run away.

Watch all the deaths around you mount...
But make like it's all fine.
Go mourn in private, silent grief,
Drown feelings with more wine.

Don't scream about how wrong this is,
Wives, mothers, daughters... DEAD!
Don't stand with others roaring... NO!!!!
Just put that past to bed.

Those women you have grown to love,
It's not like they're 'REAL' friends.
No longer empathise, support...
Right to their bitter ends.

Forget your battle, treatment's done!
It's time to end that fight.
They're telling you, you must move on.
Get on with it alright!

So carry on regardless eh,
And ditch humanity.
Plug back into the main frame now,
To keep THEIR sanity...

Edwina Maria Thompson
© 2018

NO MORE CANDLES

24th June 2018

Russian Roulette

Yet again, I am lighting another candle and raising another glass of wine. I have lost count how of many times I have done this now, and it never gets any easier.

I am a part of another family of warriors from all over the world, alongside my own tribe. These are women I will continue to stand by until my dying day: even if that is decades away. These candles we light represent the loss of lives, real lives- the loss of mothers, daughters, wives, sisters, nieces, aunts, warriors and friends. This disease Triple Negative Breast Cancer is a bastard and this is the brutal fact of the matter. If you wish to find support from ladies in the same boat as you, be it online or through 'chemo buddies' you make: then there will ultimately be deaths. Cancer KILLS and there is no nice, pink or fluffy way to explain that. Women and men out there, (including me) are losing friends, real friends. Friends who held our hands in our deepest, darkest moments; who told us- 'You can do this, just keep on fighting!' This is not just a pink heart, a pretty ribbon, a lottery or a lucky dip... this is Russian fucking Roulette for every single one of us.

Am I angry? Yeah I am, because most people just don't give a shit about cancer- not until it hits them or their families. (I was one of those once, and I am holding my hands up to this.) So many walk around with blinkers on, wallpaper over the cracks- just get on with it. I want people to see and realise how precious their life is, how f**king lucky they are to wake up only having to worry about money, mortgages, holidays or work and to not have to make the decisions women are making all over the world: whether to tell their small children they are dying; whether to try that last chemo even though nothing has worked; whether to bring forward a wedding as there is no more time; whether to take the chemotherapy while you are carrying your unborn child or wait... Could you make those decisions? Could you have the strength and resilience to keep on fighting when all else has failed? Would you rather moan at the traffic to work?

I'm sorry that I am so angry, but there are times when I think anger is the only emotion which is going to create change. We need to be angry. We need to say 'enough is enough'. We need to say "NO FUCKING MORE!"

So please I beg of you today, send a prayer to all of those ladies and men that have been have lost to this evil disease, and especially to their families and friends who are left behind to grieve each and every day.

28ᵗʰ June 2018

The Suitcases

Today I went to see the beautiful Linda Mair for some Reiki and healing. I have visited Linda before, after the death of a close friend and it was ironic that it was Linda I again needed-after another loss.

My time with Linda was wonderful (I thank you so much!). We did my cards which spoke to me clearly about the path I was on and how I had some major decisions ahead of me to make. (I'm thinking this is about my work- do I find that part time job in Costa I've always said I wanted or do I choose to write that book?) They also showed me how cherished and safe I was with those who loved me; it was comforting to know I was in a good place in that respect.

Linda also taught me a technique to help me deal with the stresses I had experienced. She asked me to imagine 2 suitcases, and I was to put all of my worries and grief into them. I was to imagine carrying these around with me (we need to learn to carry some of our experiences, rather than just let them go); but to put them down when they felt too heavy. This I was able to do.

So, I imagined I had 2 suitcases: one small purple one and one large pink one. I immediately realised that the small purple one represented my past hurts and traumas, but the large pink one was the 'Cancer' one: the one for here and now. It struck me, that despite huge amounts of pain in my past- I saw this as only small. Even my depression of 2009/10 was of little significance. (Also choosing purple represented me as it's my favourite colour.) Yet the larger suitcase, the 'Cancer' one (pink for obvious reasons I guess) - was huge.

Cancer had actually hit me harder than I had ever appreciated- it was massive in comparison to my past. Subsequently, the weight of it right now was unbearable. I had to put it down. As Linda gave me Reiki, and my thoughts and feelings emerged, I was able to process them. Some were placed in the purple suitcase- I was fine carrying these for now; and some were placed into the pink suitcase- these were not burdens I was fit enough to carry as yet.

I found this visualisation wonderful to use but it also told me a lot about myself. I was not to underestimate where I was here and now, I just had to accept that it was all too much for me at the moment. However, there would come a time when I would be able carry all of these experiences and hurts. A time would come when my strength returned, and I would be able to carry everything effortlessly. Just as I had been doing before cancer took over.

I think the reason I love this little visualisation the most- is that my lessons remain with me. I carry them, I live with them and I learn from them. Thank you yet again Linda.

29th June 2018

This time last year, I was ringing that chemotherapy bell. The only way I can describe having chemotherapy, is being taken to the edge of death and being pulled back just in time. I look back at the photo I took that morning and I see the Warrior I became staring back at me- ready to face her last battle with the little strength she had left. But I also see someone happy, someone stripped of her identity yes- but breathing, smiling, happy and free.

I didn't do any of it on my own, I had many hands behind me, around me, holding me up and carrying me at times. And to all of those who did that- I cannot ever thank them enough. I am humbled by such kindness, compassion and empathy. I was given strength and determination to fight, when I needed it the most.

So today I woke up with the biggest smile on my face. A year since the end of chemotherapy, wow! Again I looked in the mirror- make up free, chemo line gone, crazy bed hair, no baldness but this year, a tan! I still see the Warrior, this one who has lost a friend along the way. And yes my heart continues to bleed for her every day. I will never forget. But here I am today, a year on: still breathing; still smiling; still happy and still free.

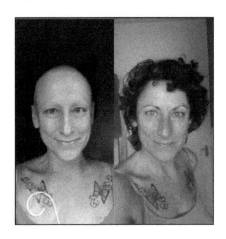

30th June 2018

This afternoon I'm going to a party and I've bought a new dress to celebrate a year from ringing that bell, but it is not the kind I would ever have bought before cancer! I am now in a place where I will dress for me, not to fit in with the crowd or to impress anyone. I even have a flower in my hair- because I want to. It is amazing how much confidence and a sense of complete freedom I have gained from losing my hair, my health and for a while there- my identity. This is a confidence I've never had, but along with it comes a deep feeling of gratitude that I'm still here to benefit from it. They say good things come to those who wait, and I have waited long enough.

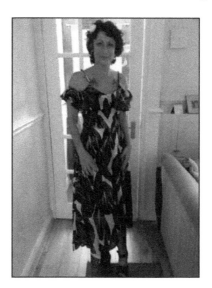

3rd July 2018

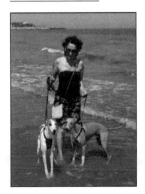

I am having a lovely time in Llandudno. This is the third year on the trot I've returned here. (I spent many years here as I went to boarding school in Rhos on Sea- a whole other story!) Last year I was in scarves and wigs to cover my head and I had drawn on eyebrows, but still so excited to be collecting Neo after the holiday. The year before, I was oblivious as to why I was losing so much weight and that cancer was already lurking. This year I'm discovering the world of frizz and have introduced Neo and Sheru to the sea! Unbelievably all of this has happened in less than 2 years. Everything constantly changes and evolves in my life and I embrace it all- whatever it brings.

4th July 2018

I was drawn recently to a memory I had as a child when I was writing an essay in History. The teacher was most put out because my character died at the end of my story, but I had written in the first person. She said that my story didn't make sense, because my character wasn't alive by the end. In my head, I had simply written from the point of view of a spirit- I didn't see the problem with this.

I've been thinking a lot about Julie and other angels we've lost. I just felt that there was more for her/them I had to get down. I like to believe every angel gets to say goodbye before they move on- wherever it is they go to. I wanted to give them the chance to come back home and say a last goodbye, even if it was only in my rose tinted imagination. And I especially like to think, that they were all there waiting for Julie when she passed on. So she was never alone.

Last Goodbyes

I tip-toed lightly round each room,
 I knew they wouldn't know.
At mirrors I just stopped and stared,
 No image did they show.
The angels had prepared me for,
 The sorrow and heartache.
A sombre grief held in the air,
 That lingered from my wake.

The vacuum here laid bare to me,
 This hole I'd left behind.
The fallout from their sudden loss.
 A cancer's curse unkind.
My final hours on earth were cruel,
 So little could I say.
And death became a welcome end,
 Too much was their dismay.

But blessed I'd been to have them there,
 All gathered by my side.
I heard each word, I saw each tear,
 As angels came to guide.
I wished I'd had the strength to say,
 No longer was I scared.
While angels gathered round my loves,
 Their soothing song I heard.

My death was gentle as a breeze,
 The angels made it so.
Warrior friends to take my hands,
 That other place to go.
I turned my thoughts to here and now,
 The past too fresh and raw.
I needed now to kiss their cheeks,
 My children whom I bore.

I climbed the stairs, I held the rail,
A tender treasured touch.
Those little things, the creaks and groans,
This home I missed so much.
The first goodbye, my daughter's room,
Heart beating now so fast.
This precious moment froze in time,
It's worth was unsurpassed.

A spirit now, so light and free,
Beside her bed, I knelt.
Curled up, asleep, her dog close by,
My broken heart did melt.
I swept the hair back from her face,
To kiss her tear stained cheek.
Then suddenly, my heart it leapt,
From slumber did she speak...

"I miss you mum, so much each day",
I wept to hear her voice.
To squeeze her tightly in my arms...
I wished I had that choice.
I kissed her hair and wiped her tears,
Her final lullaby.
Then softly crept towards the door,
I still had more goodbyes...

Her brother's room, the 'teenage den',
His haven from this mess.
A space he blitzed just once a week
Enough for him I guess...
Yet in the doorway, there I saw,
A space to make me proud.
To help his dad and 'do his bit',
My precious boy had vowed.

Lay on his back, with tiny snores,
If only he could hear.
I'd tell him how much pride I felt,
My smile from ear to ear.
Again I knelt beside the bed,
To kiss his sleepy brow.
These precious chances for goodbyes,
All paused in time somehow.

Soon I knew, the moment had come,
The last goodbye to make.
My one true love, my rock, my strength,
Whose heart I'd had to break...
If only I could hold him now,
And vanquish all despair.
Then whisper to him, 'It's ok,
I'm free now, as the air.'

Lovingly lay along his side,
So close I felt his breath.
Nothing now to separate us,
An oath beyond my death.
No longer was I body here,
Just spirit in the night.
But still the love I held for him,
As boundless as starlight.

Our noses touched, his nostrils twitched,
A kiss placed on my lips.
Instinctively he'd sensed me there,
My heart was beating skips.
Memories spun throughout my mind,
The times we'd lay like this.
Despite the cancer, tears and pain,
Were moments of pure bliss.

To stay forever... never leave,
If only that could be.
But everything in time must pass,
No-one lives endlessly...
I'd lived my life with no regrets,
With laughter, love and fun.
Those angel kisses, left behind,
Our last goodbyes were done.

Edwina Maria Thompson
© 2018

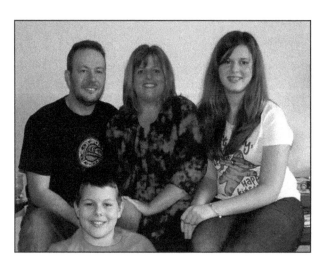

13th July 2018

We had another meet up today for the warriors. It was only me and Cath to begin with, but I'm glad to say that Joanne managed to join us last minute. Neither of us had seen Jo since Julie died, so today was quite a difficult one. I went through Julie's last weeks and days, trying to make some sort of sense of it for Jo- as to how she had passed away so quickly and suddenly. There was no easy way to convey what happened and the three of us sat in tears as we remembered her. I think Jo has done incredibly well to hold herself together with everything, especially as she is still undergoing her treatments. It was only due to chemotherapy day that she couldn't make the funeral. We still managed some laughter though and Jo said how she has bought a sunflower for her garden. It put the biggest smile on my face, knowing that Julie can still bring the sunshine. Another sad meet up yes, but I know they will become easier in time.

14th July 2018

There are so many reasons that draw me to writing and I love it when I get to write for one of our own warriors. This poem has been written for our wonderful young warrior Emma Knowles. She is battling hard against her cancer, and is constantly a source of love, light and hope to us all in our group. (It was Emma who spoke so passionately in a blog on Triple Negative Awareness Day.) The spirit of this young lady inspires me every day. *#ourqueenbeeswish*

Emma's Wish

I first knew Emma through our group,
All fighting this disease.
A Wonder Woman in our midst,
A "Queen Bee" with such breeze!

Her battle took her to the depths,
A hell no girl should face.
Yet Queen Bee has stood tall and strong,
She's fought with charm and grace.

Her battle now has done it's worst,
She knows her days are short.
And yet she still smiles on with hope,
But asks for your support...

Her one true wish now is to meet,
Her idol...Beyonce!
So we are tweeting, sharing, fast...
To grant her wish one day!

We beg of you to help us now,
To get our message through!
So Tweet or share, for our Queen Bee!!
Please make her wish come true.

Edwina Maria Thompson
© 2018

18th July 2018

Not particularly worried, but I know I'm going to have to monitor this. In the last week or so, I've had a few episodes where I've gone very dizzy- room spinning, eye sight blurred and on the verge of passing out. It's not gone straight away and takes about 30 seconds or so for me to feel normal again. Most times it's happened I've been sitting down, and have just turned my head or been turning around. So it can't be from standing up too quickly. Alongside that, I'm having crushing headaches in the night. I think if it doesn't improve, I'm going back to the doctors. (They'll be sick of me but what else are you meant to do?) I've got a boil that isn't clearing either, so maybe a phone call to the Breast Cancer nurse would be a better idea? The worry never really goes away. Finding the balance between being cautious, vigilant and sensible without becoming a hypochondriac is not easy!

HIPPO DAYS AND HAPPY DAYS

19th July 2018

Hippo Days and Happy Days

In the last week or so, I've seen lots of people I haven't seen in a while and it was lovely. It really is fab being told how well you look, I'll not deny that. However, the harsh reality of this disease, the destructive treatments and the aftermath- is that people only ever actually see us at our best. After a ridiculously busy week last week, (in my terms, not a fit persons) it took me three days to recover. Then today, after only one busy day- I'm floored again.

This is me right now: a swollen face from a headache all night; fatigue that's drained me making just climbing the stairs a chore; pain in my joints, hands, feet, knees and hips; and still grieving heavily for my beautiful friend.

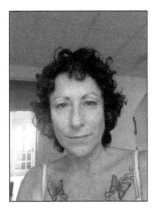

This is our reality, we have to find a way to carry it all. This is how we live afterwards, but we often only ever show you the healthy face and not the truth. Just as we covered our baldness and loss of our image with a wig and make up- we show you what you want to see: that cancer isn't the shit, soul destroying hell that people are scared of and that it can be beaten. The truth is, cancer is with you for many, many years and recovery doesn't happen in a few months because that can take years too. Today, I can't carry it, it's just too much. I have to put it down for my own health and sanity. I will recharge, reset and have a 'Hippo Day'. So tomorrow I can fight again and hopefully it can be a 'Happy day'.

So please, if you know someone out there who is recovering from cancer, the loss of a loved one or any difficulty/trauma in their lives (even years down the line); then maybe ask the question- "How are you truly, behind it all?" No matter how well they look. Sometimes, as I said once in a poem- this is how we actually are...

'So next time you see me,
With 'wisdom' to share...
Remember I'm struggling,
With just being there.'

22ⁿᵈ July 2018

So today is a pretty special day for me. I am returning to teaching a Yoga workshop, after 18 months. It is a huge step for me, teaching in this way is mentally and emotionally challenging; but the students gain so much and I absolutely love it.

My theme is 'Love and Faith'. I chose a story about Hanuman, a Hindu Monkey god who is celebrated and worshipped for his undying devotion and his selfless dedication to his friend Rama. Hanuman is the son of the wind god Vayu, but has no memory of his childhood and thus has no idea that he is half divine. His strength and courage come from his love for his friend, and this is a story which touches my heart in so many ways. I chose it for all of the warriors I have grown to love, as it shows how, sometimes, we can forget our own strength, bravery and fortitude- that we are actually our own 'hero'. We simply forget to have faith in ourselves.

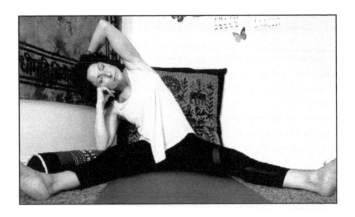

24th July 2018

There are so many feelings you experience on your journey
with cancer. Some days are good, some days are hard and
some days are just hell on earth. In looking back, I've come to
call my good days, 'Happy Days', my sadder days 'Hippo
Days' and the most brutal, the 'Hero Days'.

The first Hero Day was the day we shaved my head. I'd had
long hair, so to become bald was a huge deal. When you do
begin to lose your hair, it hurts- it's really painful when it
comes out. So often, people will take control and shave it
beforehand. This was what I did. I'll not lie, it's devastating-
but liberating too. YOU choose to shave it, not cancer.

Once it was shaved I looked in the mirror and I saw a warrior,
ready to do battle. My strength soared; I knew I could do
ANYTHING! Then I took a picture and I literally was on fire,
my aura was ablaze. There was my 'patronus' (yes, I am very
much a Harry Potter fan). Just as Harry realises the one who
saves him and Sirius by the lake- is actually his future self.
I realised, my Patronus charm was within- it was me.

Hero Days

I am my own Hero,
I've come to realise.
Phoenix, wolf, warrior...
All three are my disguise.

I fought through many wars,
Being cut, poisoned, burnt.
Each one, in it's own way,
With lessons to be learnt.

In dark days of treatment,
You sink into the mire.
Wading your way through it,
Is all that you desire.

You're drowning in darkness,
A labyrinth of hell.
No light there to guide you,
Just tolling of death's knell.

But somehow then, she grows,
The hero deep within.
With sword and shield held high,
Your battle does begin.

I saw my hero rise,
In shaving off my hair.
Looking in the mirror,
My courage clearly there.

No need to wave a wand,
Protective spells to cast.
There was my 'patronus',
A hero unsurpassed.

An aura around me,
My spirit now ablaze.
Fired up and ready,
For savage Hero Days.

Hero Days are brutal,
You cannot hide from that.
They bring you to your knees,
In punishing combat.

But time then makes of you,
A warrior of old.
Battle scared... but Hero,
Your crusade to be told.

Edwina Maria Thompson
© 2018

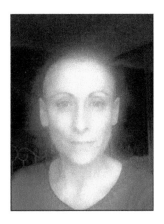

1st August 2018

I have come to the conclusion that I am in a very silly mood today. Hoping this is some of my usual personality returning after being so effing knackered- woo hoo if it is! Long may it last? Maybe it's the decision to ditch the medication for neuropathy (it has made me gain weight, crave sugary foods and made me lethargic) and opt for anything else that'll help instead- yoga, turmeric, cod liver oil, bee pollen, starflower oil, ginseng, vitamin d3, anything! Hopefully it's going to help joint pain, back pain, peripheral neuropathy, arthritis, fatigue, menopause, hot flushes and insomnia. Wow Cancer, you do like to leave your little 'gifts' don't you?

3rd August 2018

So today, I went back to the Breast Clinic about the headaches I've been getting and the boil on my side. The nurse takes my blood pressure and I sit there with a pretty smug look on my face, telling her how most of my family have high blood pressure: but I don't. Even through treatments it wasn't high! (Hmmm, is that ego there again Edwina?) She turns to me and said the last thing I was expecting- well it's high today. Oh My God, me with high blood pressure? You are having a laugh!

She let me calm down for a while (I was not happy) and took it again- still high. With two parents having coronary heart disease and both going through a Triple Bypass, this is not what I wanted to know. I can remember my brother asking my mum how bad the operation was when we visited her in hospital. I couldn't understand why he wanted to know that; so I said, 'Why are you asking her that?' 'Well' he says, 'law of probability, one of us is bound to need one.'- nothing like being positive eh? I'm already in the 'Cancer' camp', do I really have to be in another camp too?

5th August 2018

The Hangover

I'm currently lying in bed nursing a hangover (that should be considerably worse than it is!) Last night Lynn and I went out for a drink, like we used to of old. I can't begin to say how much we laughed; we really had the best time. I know I am not my old self anymore and that's ok, but I do have a new me I think- better, sillier, funnier, and dafter. The night was absolutely hilarious and for the whole night I didn't think once about cancer! I attempted to dance the way I used to (you gotta try eh); but my knees just wouldn't allow me. This did mean I got stuck on numerous occasions in ridiculous dance moves, with Lynn then having to help me back up. It was like watching one of Anton's partners on Strictly- I was more like a cart horse than a Darcy. (And to think a student once asked me if I'd been a ballerina, so much for that now!) At one point we had to sit down because I was exhausted. Suddenly I felt myself slipping under the table off my chair and that was before I'd even had too much. I could tell this was going to be an eventful night!

Later in the night, we met a lovely guy who knew of me through my yoga and cancer journey. I had taught his wife's friend who is also going through cancer treatment; it is so wonderful how cancer has allowed me to reach out to many more people in need. He bought us both drinks to say thank you and I was really touched by such a kind gesture from someone I didn't even know. By the end of the night though, I was in a lot of pain, (unfortunately I can't cope with heels as well as I used to.) So Lynn talked a taxi guy who was booked for someone else, into driving us home. (She's a goodun.) A good night had been had by us both by all accounts. It truly felt like old times.

When we got back to mine at 3am however, we discovered I'd forgotten my key. Absolutely typical, you can't take me anywhere! It was one of those moments when you can't control yourself. I was laughing so much about it, I couldn't throw a stone at the window to wake my partner. I raised my arm to throw it but it fell backwards out of my hand onto the floor. I tried again and the same thing happened, so that was it then. I fell into a heap of hysteria! How I didn't wet myself I don't know. Lynn was stood there saying- 'Just give me the bloody stone!' In this madness I staggered over to a parked car and tried to lean up against it. Tears were streaming down my face with laughter as I slowly slid down the side of the car I was leaning on, in complete stitches at the sight of Lynn trying to throw the stone instead. I'll be honest- I don't even know or remember how we got in!

Then we come to this morning of course. I woke up with a blinding headache, as you can imagine- so I decided paracetamol was in need. In my hung over state or maybe still drunk to be honest- I tried to slide down the stairs on my belly to get the paracetamol: simply because I couldn't stand up. Yes, there is still much of the old Edwina in me! I might add, I did creep in to see how Lynn was doing, and she's not much better than me. Nice to know I'm not the only one suffering. Our love for Captain Morgan's Spiced Rum hasn't withered then! Yep, I am definitely back on form- kind of anyway!

Last night was amazing. It reminded me how truly lucky I am- with everything and everyone I have. A crazy but fantastic friend (and others!) who have stood by me throughout, a boyfriend who picks me up time and again when I hit a brick wall, my mum who messages me often that I'm in her prayers, a body that still works most of the time, two beautiful girls, a roof over my head, a warm bed, running water, two gorgeous dogs who love me unconditionally... need I go on?

Life is too short, it's not a cliché, it's true. I've seen the best and worst of people in the last 18 months and I've seen the best and worst of myself. I'm not perfect at all but I never claim to be. I'm impatient, lazy sometimes, selfish but then I have other incredible qualities too. I laugh and I cry. I'm human.

This month I'm cutting back, I'm taking a time out. I'm remembering to live. The appointment I had at the hospital on

Friday really gave me a head's up. As I said, I've been having bizarre headaches, blurred vision, dizziness, and a boil which hasn't cleared. So, the result is, the cyst is going to be removed, and I'm getting a CT brain scan. (Yes, they may well not find a brain, I know!) This is the first time, (even though it's hopefully only a cyst and the headaches are possibly just menopause) -that my instincts aren't sure. I don't know what's in store; I have no idea how to feel. None. On one hand I'm positive everything is 100% fine -on the other hand I remain prepared in case it isn't. Triple Negative is a bastard and I am only too aware of that. There are no hard or fast rules with it, it is a game of Russian Roulette and I'm playing it whether I choose to or not.

Last night, I got pissed; I acted like a fool in every pub. I remembered to live! Life really is too short. Stop and smell the flowers, dance in the rain, find those rainbows, because you won't be here forever. That's your only guarantee of which you can be absolutely sure.

6th August 2018

It was being in my Triple Negative Warrior UK group, which first inspired me to write. So many of the poems are about me, but some are about other ladies with TN, and of course some are about Julie.

I've written so often of the difficult times of cancer because at the end of the day, it is like a hell on earth. But I do believe that it gives you something else -gratitude for your life, health and happiness. Yes, I've had many Hippo Days and Hero Days I'd rather forget; but here they are at last- the 'Happy Days'. And they are coming more and more frequently as the months roll on by. This is for anyone who is just beginning their journey with cancer; in the hope, that one day, your Happy Days do come too.

Happy Days

Today will be a Happy Day,
I feel it in my bones.
A smile has spread across my face.
Forget my aches and groans!

I'll rise right up, leap out of bed,
And throw those curtains wide!
To thank the dawn for this new day,
Let life be a joyride!

I'll greet my puppies, play around,
Act like I'm still a kid!
Cram all of life into this day.
(My last one? God forbid!)

I'll soak in everything I see,
Appreciate small things.
I'll cherish moments 'here and now',
My rising heart, it springs!

I'll compliment the friends I see,
And loving kindness send.
Be mindful of each breath I take,
My gratitude transcends.

I'll smell those flowers, dance in rain,
Find rainbows in the sky.
Meet with friends for coffee and cake.
And watch the world go by.

I'll take my time, a gentle pace.
Just as Italians say...
Sweetly to do... nothing at all.
"Dolce far niente."

I'll focus more on what I say,
A 'thank-you' goes so far.
Remember those who stood by me,
Then thank my lucky stars!

And yes my thoughts will drift to those...
Whose spirits still, I feel.
I'll offer days like this, to them...
And honour life with zeal.

I won't forget this 'Happy Day',
I see them more and more...
And yes, I swear, they all make up,
For Hippo Days I bore.

Edwina Maria Thompson
© 2018

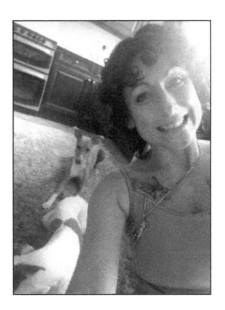

7th August 2018

Finally went for the colonic I've been promising myself and my belly is flat again! Yey! All I have to do now is tone up again. I highly recommend one but at least 3 months after treatment is all done. I go to Balance Health Centre in Tuebrook, Liverpool. Allison is absolutely fab!

10th August 2018

Well, 18 months from diagnosis and there she is. Let me introduce you to Edwina the yogini, the girl who draws a sun on her 3rd eye- because she wants too. For the first time tonight, I truly saw her again, in me. Only she's a little feistier than the first one! Never in a million years did I ever feel like I would get my yoga mojo back- but here it is. Don't be fooled by the poses though, the true part of my yoga spirit actually lies within.

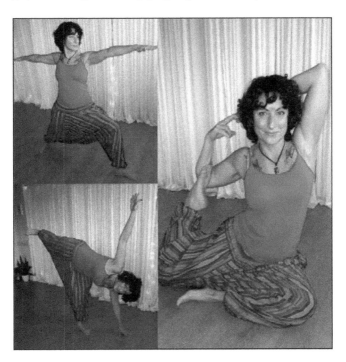

SO I BEGIN AGAIN

13th August 2018

Triple Negative Breast Cancer

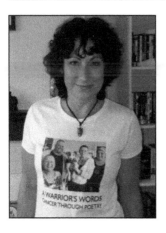

My t-shirt for A Warrior's Words has arrived! I am currently putting together my poems, blogs and diary into a format so they can all be published. As the whole process needs time, editing and formatting, I'm still a way yet from an actual book. I'm hoping it will take less time than I expect though. Poetry has also become my yoga of recent months and if you actually study the Yoga Sutras, you will find that 'asana' (poses) are only a fraction of the practice of yoga itself. So that mine has evolved to include writing, is not a surprise.

This book is not just to raise awareness for Triple Negative Breast Cancer but in memory of my beautiful friend Julie who sadly was taken by this cruel and brutal disease. It is also in memory of the many other ladies who have been lost: mums, sisters, daughters, wives, aunties, nieces- none of whom should have died. My poems have come not just from my own experiences, but from many other women I have been blessed to know and love.

So what is Triple Negative Breast Cancer? Why has no one heard of it? I sure as hell hadn't. Surely all breast cancers are the same? Absolutely not. Breast cancer is usually fuelled by oestrogen or progesterone (hormones), or HER2 (a growth protein). Triple Negative is so called as it tests negative for these three growth receptors. In each of these other hormone/protein positive cases, the cancers can be given a targeted treatment or hormone therapy. This basically means, they can block the action of whatever it is that is fueling the growth of the cancer cells. (Obviously, I am in no way suggesting these breast cancers are 'better' to have; simply that some have a tried and tested treatment.) Unfortunately in these cases, it also means that the targeted treatments do have to be taken for years. Whereas with Triple Negative, once we pass the 5 year mark- we are pretty much clear: our chances of recurrence or the cancer having spread drop to a minimal. There is absolutely a positive in the negative!

Regards treatments for Triple Negative Breast Cancer (TNBC for short), there is NO targeted treatment and no long term medication to keep it at bay. You are given all they can offer- surgery, chemotherapy and radiotherapy- which are all very aggressive treatments for the body. They hit it with the works and blast you to oblivion to give you the best chance of survival. But it doesn't end there. TNBC has a higher recurrence rate (in laymen's terms, it could return even after it's been cut out). It also has a higher chance of spreading to the rest of the body. If this happens, you are only treatable and no longer curable. In the case of Stage 4, (metastatic cancer that has spread to other parts of the body), you are then classed as terminal. This is the case for ALL cancers- you become a 'cancer lifer'. This is not a term many would want to use and obviously in an aggressive TN diagnosis- it can be terrifying. However with so much research being done into TN and the many trials taking place, I know that prognosis is definitely improving!

TNBC is a bastard, it took Julie and that is the only name it deserves. It takes with no rhyme nor reason and it has no hard or fast rules to it. We all carry the same chances, we're all in the same 'Lucky Dip' and it takes the young more often than not. They know it also linked to family history and our genes. So far they have found many genes related to TNBC, the most commonly known being BRCA1 and 2. I wish I knew if I was one of those carrying the gene so I could be monitored and my daughters and family could be tested. If myself, or more importantly my daughters have the gene, huge decisions would have to be made. In many cases, a double mastectomy and removal of ovaries is recommended. Unfortunately my NHS trust won't test me, despite NICE guidelines saying I should 'automatically' be tested with TNBC as I am under 50 years of age. So much of treatment and care in the NHS boils down to your postcode, and I'm obviously in the wrong one! It is what it is, but one day I think we will all be genetically tested for common diseases as a matter of course. Let's hope that day isn't too far in the future.

So I push in my own little way to raise awareness of Triple Negative Breast Cancer but also to help raise more funds for research into TN. Please God, one day may they find a cure for each and every one.

14th August 2018

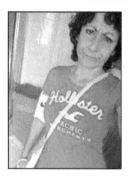

I have to admit I was a tad pissed off this afternoon. I went for my 24 hour blood pressure monitor and it was effing high again. I know in the whole scheme of things it's nothing really; but I did think I had escaped the family curse. Maybe I spoke too soon? Unfortunately, coronary heart disease did eventually kill my father, but luckily my mum is still with us. I do know that her surgeon said her arteries were tiny and so it made the operation a nightmare to do. My dad's arteries were wide, hence him lasting 20 odd years before it actually killed him at 61. (So my brother says). When I went for my Hickman line last year, the nurse actually said, 'Oh no, your veins are so tiny.' Brilliant that's all I needed to know!

So my latest accessory for the next 24 hours is a blood pressure monitor to check what's going on. It feels like my arm's gonna fall off every time it goes up so I'm chanting away in my head each time- 'Oooommmmm.'

15th August 2018

Oh my god, well I think I've heard it all now! This is a conversation I had this morning with one of the 'younger generation'. It took a lot of deep breathing not to react.

Y: Life is a race. If you don't get there first, you lose.

Me: (laughing) No it isn't.

Y: Yes it is; you race until you die.

Me: OK. You've got a lot to learn about life then...

Y: No I don't. You've got a lot to learn about death.

Me: (a little stunned at that one, as my past is known well enough): I think I stared death in the face a few times in the last 18 months.

Y: Well you obviously didn't learn enough about it then did you!

I left it there and decided to walk away calmly. I'm very impressed that I kept my gob shut! There again, I don't know where other people's paths have taken them do I?

19th August 2018

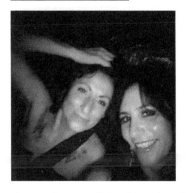

Last night I went out for Lynn's 50th in Chester. I'd been a bit apprehensive because I've not been so far for an all-day 'do' since diagnosis. I rested the day before, then only had 1 drink and paced myself. But I also thought, f**k it I'm dressing like I used to in my 30s! I had an absolute ball and at the end of the night- I still had loads of energy. How amazing is that? We were still having a ball on the mini bus home. It is true, even though you never think it will happen- you really do get a lot of 'you' back.

18- 19th August 2018

I have wanted to write a poem for Julie's yoga mat for a while, and the room I made for us to do yoga together. I have taken to using her mat to teach on now. It goes with me to every class and has become my haven of safety. There are times when I wish I could have taught her, just once- but that was never meant to be. We did get to go to a class together, though, and I cherish that time we had. Even Cath said recently at the end of my class, she wished that Julie could have experienced the feeling of contentment that she gets from yoga. In reality though, there was very little I could ever have done to help.

<u>The Yoga Mat</u>

I have your yoga mat now, my dear friend.
It was passed on to me when you died.
Over weeks, I did nothing... but lie there,
A safe place, for the tears that I cried.

I would sing in my head, many mantra,
And believe you could hear every note.
The smiles would creep across a teared face,
As your memories kept me afloat.

I'd imagine, I'd been blessed to teach you,
That I'd helped you, to cope with your pain.
Picturing poses we did side by side,
With some peace, that I'd hoped you'd attain.

Looking around, at this space that I made,
So inspired by all of your needs.
Even though you, never stepped in this room,
I still feel, it has sown many seeds.

The sweet smell of frankincense in the air,
Our poems that hang on the wall.
Butterflies, candles, Buddha, Ganesh,
And an Indian tapestry tall.

This space would never exist, without you,
As I lie on your mat to reflect.
Every lesson I teach now, you're there,
That I take you with me, is perfect.

And maybe your mat, was never rolled out,
But I do that for you every day.
I look to the future, breathe in the 'now',
Let the past remain in, yesterday.

Yes, my dear friend... your yoga mat is mine.
You are an 'instructor honouree'
I promise I'll never, leave you behind,
As together we teach harmony.

Your spirit will be in every word,
Loving kindness is what I'll impart.
May each of my lessons, honour your life.
Let them radiate hope, from my heart.

Edwina Maria Thompson
© 2018

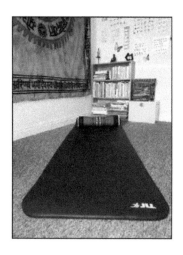

20th August 2018

Today I have had the best time with Katya at Lotusflower Yoga Studio doing a yoga video together. It is lovely to work alongside another instructor and you can't partner with a lovelier lady than Katya! We had such a laugh and even though we had to film twice, it just made it better. We make a fab double act too; you'd think we were a comedy duo. Katya has become my yoga instructor of recent years and the support and love she has given me is wonderful. This little lady is getting me back to health and she even got me in a handstand! You can find our video on the Lotusfloweryoga YouTube Channel. It is called Yoga for Cancer.

22nd August 2018

There is a wonderful lady in our Triple Negative group who has been given the worst news recently- that the cancer has spread to her brain. It couldn't be more devastating for her, as she has a little girl she just wants to be there for. There is no way to describe the unfairness in young mums being diagnosed with stage 4 and often in this country the treatment just isn't good enough. She is fighting a battle not only for her own life, but for her little girl, her husband and her family. This is Jade's story.

Just Jade

Raise my little girl is all, I simply want to do.
Watch her face light up in awe, when she learns something new...
Snuggle up in bed with books, to read the whole night through.
Just be Jade.

Make my mother have to run, to keep up with my pace!
Do my job as officer, protect the human race.
Not accept a treatment that, feels like it's second place...
Just be Jade.

Squeeze my husband day and night,
and keep our marriage strong.
Never have to face a time, I reach my last 'swan song'.
Grasp this chance that I may have, prognosis to prolong.
Just be Jade.

Get my cancer known out there, shout loud "TNBC!".
Triple Negative it's name, this bastard killing spree.
Striking women all too young, whose lives should be care free.
Just like Jade.

Beat this cancer, let it know, it's picked a badass foe!
Battle ready, hear me cry, my fire is aglow!
Try your best, I'll fight each breath!
That towel in, I won't throw!
I. AM. JADE!

Edwina Maria Thompson
© 2018

23rd August 2018

Well here it is: the poem I have been meaning to write for over a year and this one is for you Carole-Anne. (I got there in the end, woo hoo!) This group of women I have grown to love and respect are called Triple Negative Warriors UK and they are unstoppable! It is through this incredible group that I have met so many new friends: friends I will forever cherish, be they online or face to face. We stand tall and strong supporting each other through the highs and lows of this disease. We fight together, we laugh together, we cry together and we shout together... this is our song. HEAR OUR CRY!

TRIPLE NEGATIVE WARRIORS UK

Meet the TN Girls UK
Warriors, not cancer prey.
"TRIPLE NEGATIVE" our cry,
Wanting you to ask us WHY?

1...2...3...4,
Hear our TNBC roar!
5...6...7...8,
Raise awareness for our fate!

Mothers, daughters, sisters, wives,
Standing tall to save more lives.
Facing cancer down so rare,
Will it beat us? LET IT DARE!

1...2...3...4,
Hear our TNBC roar!
5...6...7...8,
TNBC elevate!

Diff'rent that is what we are.
All those treatments, we go far!
Not breast cancer as you think
We're a special shade of pink!

1...2...3...4,
Hear our TNBC roar!
5...6...7...8,
Raise awareness for our fate!

Fighters, we become the best,
Warriors with souls possessed.
Ever there to lend support,
Kindness that just can't be bought!

1...2...3...4,
Hear our TNBC roar!
5...6...7...8,
TNBC elevate!

Warriors we stand in line,
Blessed to have our friends so fine.
Toughest girls, who won't back down.
Wear with pride, our TN Crown!

1...2...3...4,
Hear our TNBC roar!
5...6...7...8,
Raise awareness for our fate!

Stricken fam'lies fit to burst,
Warriors who took the worst.
All our angels flying high,
In your names WE SEND OUR CRY!

1...2...3...4,
Hear our TNBC ROAR!
5...6...7...8,
TNBC ELEVATE!

Edwina Maria Thompson
© 2018

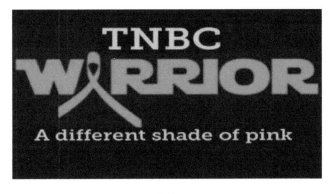

31st August 2018

Woo hoo, the results of my brain scan are back… and it's clear! Hopefully the headaches are just from my blood pressure (still not got those results yet though). They could also be from coming off my medication for neuropathy so I've been told.

I might add though, the nurse did say that my brain was 'unremarkable': brilliant eh? So it would seem that after all of these years- that my teachers were right all along!

3rd September 2018

I've just had the best news I could have wished for! I went to have my cyst removed but the surgeon has agreed it's gone now. It began to shrink in the last week so I'm made up. There is still a large mark left, but I can live with that! I've obviously got to keep an eye on it though in case it returns.

9th September 2018

This afternoon I took all of the writing I have been doing to Julie's family. It was an absolute honour to show them the poems and the diary of Julie's and my time together. We went through everything I had written about Julie, looked at the many photos I have collected, and shared so many stories. It was wonderful how they were able to fill in a few things that my chemo wrecked brain had forgotten! As her daughter Hannah said also, it's important to be honest throughout and talk about the difficult times as well as the good ones. There were quite a few poems that they hadn't heard or read. So every poem about her, I read to them. I can't begin to express how powerful it was for us all. Colin, Julie's dad said something beautiful to me, 'Not only will the poems keep Julie's spirit alive for us; they will help others on this journey too.'

They were also able to give me some photos of Julie and them all together, to use with her poems. As I drove home, I found it so overwhelming. I can only hope I am able to help others on this path and that I can let people know about the amazing lady that was Julie Ainsworth. I feel truly honoured to be doing this in her memory.

14th September 2018

Today has been pretty special, my 49th birthday. I am so utterly excited about the fact that I will be 50 next time! It seems incredible after the last 18 months that hitting 50 looks like a probability now. Nothing is going to get in my way I hope, certainly not cancer. I might add though, I have decided to start my celebrations this year- why the hell not? So I have made myself a long list of things I want to do this coming year: a visit to Harry Potter World, dancing lessons like Strictly, a hot–air balloon ride, getting up close with elephants at Chester Zoo, taking a picnic on a hill, eating fish and chips on the prom at Blackpool Illuminations, a visit to Llandudno again... my list goes on. How often do we wait around for special occasions to 'do' things? Well, I'm not waiting! It begins right now. Why on earth do I have to wait until my 50th year to make special memories? It's not a 'Bucket List' either, because I don't intend to kick any bucket any time soon! It is a 'Life List'. I am choosing to live and not to worry my life away wondering 'what if'. I want to live for now and not for tomorrow.

So today, I fulfilled another of my Living List wishes- I went out for a birthday meal with my beautiful girls. I had an amazing time and yet again managed to get a photo with them. Long may the traditional Birthday Photo continue... until I am old and grey and they are too.

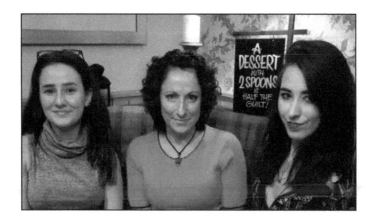

20th September 2018

Recently I have been listening to a particular Yoga Nidra that I downloaded from the Internet. Back in January, I went on a course to study this form of meditation/relaxation a little more in depth. The course itself was run by the Yoga Nidra Network, and it is a meditation called 'Fertile Darkness' delivered by Fiona Law that I have been listening to on their website. Each time I listened, I fell asleep. No big surprise as it does last 40 minutes, but I knew there was something important being said to me. So today, I forced myself to stay awake and listen (and not just let my subconscious do all the work!) I was both intrigued and inspired by what was said.

Fiona talks of a 'fertile darkness'- a dark soil where there lies an 'irrepressible force of regeneration'. It reminded me of a forest after a wild fire, burnt to the ground with that black seemingly barren darkness. She calls it 'fertile warmth', a place where life can begin to grow again, as of course it always does. We know that even after the worst bush fires, life will eventually spring forth- nothing can stop it. 'Life will always find a way' (a quote from Jurassic Park!) It is that darkest of soils where everything lies in waiting, waiting for the dormancy to end and the new life to begin: as Fiona describes it- 'the hint of

236

life from underground.' Then it struck me: this is where I am-in this Fertile Darkness lying dormant, waiting for my regeneration to take hold. It is my place of safety and warmth, a place to hibernate and rejuvenate ready for a new beginning and a new life. I understand that totally, it makes absolute sense. And so yet another piece falls into place.

29th September 2018

Julie's Coffee Morning

Today has been a wonderful day. Last year, Julie had wanted to arrange a Coffee Morning on her birthday but hadn't had the chance to do so. (She had a fab weekend away instead!) This year, her mum, brother and family held that event for her, in her memory. Shirley has been baking like a mad woman for days to prepare for it, and it couldn't have been more successful. She has managed to raise £421 for the Shine Bright Foundation and everyone is delighted that so much was raised! I have no doubt that Julie is smiling down, incredibly proud at the hard work that has taken place.

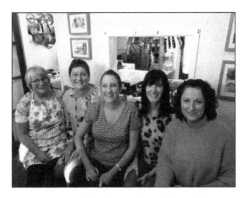

I invited some of the Triple Negative ladies too, so it was lovely to meet more ladies that had connected with Julie. The whole house was full and I don't think I have ever seen so many cakes in one house. Deb was hilarious today, checking that the cakes were completely calorie free before she ate them. (Of course they were Deb.) Calories don't count when it's for charity anyway. I had two slices of salted caramel cheesecake and it was delicious! Cath was there with

Shelly and Tracey and we got together with Shirley for a photo. You may not have been there in body Julie, but you were there in spirit. What a memorable day, and one that I think is going to be an annual event. How fantastic!

1st October 2018

So I Begin Again

And so I begin again- a new me, a new adventure and a new challenge. I have almost completed my metamorphosis from Yoga Instructor to Cancer Patient to Poet/Author and this is the last piece of writing to end my whole journey. I am amazed at how this has become yet another passion in my life: first teaching, then yoga and now poetry and writing. I feel so incredibly blessed that the universe has chosen to lay all this at my feet: that I have the opportunity to live a different life again and to experience the world through other people's eyes. I can imagine walking in their shoes, express what this evil disease does... and then share it with the world. In many cases I've been told that I have described through my poetry what others were thinking and feeling but couldn't put it into words themselves. I am both honoured and humbled to do so and just hope that in some way these poems may allow others to understand what this disease does to people. Let them strip away the ribbons, the pink, the hearts, the fears and the myths and show cancer in it's true form: raw, cruel, brutal and heart breaking... but also what it brings: inspiration, unity, hope, courage, and of course love. I quote my guru Wendy again: 'Like a dark shadow, sometimes it leaves light.'

Personally I have never doubted throughout my journey that there was a reason I had cancer. I was one of those people who thought cancer treatment was a huge con, that the 'cure' was already there but 'big pharma' was hiding the secret away. (I had this image in my head of a huge laboratory deep underground where only an elite few had access to the 'cure'.) I smile now when I think about this. I've no doubt there is someone somewhere making an awful lot of money- there always is. But I am educated enough in my own cancer now to know that 'cancer' isn't just one disease, it's hundreds in fact. There are over 200 types of cancer I believe. Even within TN, there are 6 subtypes and so a cure is way off for every single type of cancer and their subtypes. We do need more research, we do need more money, we do need more genetic testing and we do need more awareness! So maybe one of my lessons on this journey was to become more educated and less judgemental or sceptical. I can safely say that lesson has been well and truly learnt!

I still have no idea if cancer will ultimately be the end for me, and that I accept. Statistically, I am more likely to survive TN as most of us are, but that doesn't mean that many won't. It is the cruel reality of cancer: it kills too often. However, none of us really know when our last breath will be, do we? So actually I am no different to anyone else who has never faced cancer. Like I have said on many occasions, the very fact that I am here since my first bout of depression- is a miracle. I am blessed daily with the gift of life and I am grateful for that with every ounce of my being. It takes me back to the conversations Vannessa and I used to have about life. When we used to wonder why we were experiencing so much heartache, tragedy and death. We could see how unpredictable life was and how easily everything could change in the blink of an eye. We knew that our lives were precious, that every experience was important no matter how difficult it was and we knew never to take anything for granted.

I do believe that we are only given lessons and challenges in life that we can handle, but it is those challenges and lessons that mould us and shape us. They make us who we are. It was only thanks to my original breakdown that I was able to discover yoga. I could have continued to plummet, allowed the darkness to overwhelm the light- but I didn't. I found the light again through yoga and it has been my salvation since. But yoga poses, meditation or breathing techniques aren't the answer to everyone's problems, they can't be. I have said to students on many occasions: yoga can be anything. It is whatever unites your heart, mind, body and soul- horse riding, running, drawing, even poetry. It is whatever helps us to rejuvenate our souls- not what we do on a mat. It is simply whatever we need to get us through life with that sense of 'santosha'-contentment. We can't control what happens in life, no one can, but we can control how we react and that is the crucial solution to any of our problems. I think how we react to our problems in life ultimately determines what we learn from it too. If we react to a problem with negative emotions, then that is what that problem will manifest: fear breeds fear, hatred breeds hatred, envy breeds envy etc. We see it every day in the world. Yet in exactly the same way- love breeds love, kindness breeds kindness, patience breeds patience, and empathy breeds empathy.

It is that love, kindness, patience and empathy I have seen throughout my journey and I can honestly say it has overwhelmed me. There is nothing more inspirational and moving than seeing a person battling a terminal disease offer their love, hope and energy to support another in pain. I have seen it over and over again and I remember Julie doing exactly that when she held Jo's hands in the garden centre. Now that is true humanity right there. That is one soul reaching out to guide and love another. My friend was a brave, compassionate, thoughtful and loving soul: a wonderful wife, mother, daughter, sister, aunty and friend. She was one of those special people in life who touch you in a way you can't even begin to describe and her spirit resides in so much of my work. My heart goes out to her family and friends who are lost daily without her, and I pray that her love and light shines through in my words: that they will forever be a reminder of what an inspirational lady Julie Ainsworth was and still is. If only the whole world could have a little of Julie's kindness and spirit- what an even more beautiful place it would be.

And so I begin again- from the fertile darkness that cancer has created for me. I feel like the tiniest shoot just beginning to break from the darkness into the light- a light that is exquisite. The future is unwritten for me now, but I am ready for it all- the good, the bad and even the ugly. I am embracing this new love of writing with passion and grace as it searches for an understanding of my world and purpose in life. I return to teaching my classes with a deeper empathy for others in the hope that they reach out to each and every soul that enters in. Maybe now I have finally found my 'dharma', my duty in life? Who knows? Life and all that it brings is a huge adventurous roller coaster ride, that's for sure. So I plan to sit up at the front exhilarated with the wind in my face and new hair, reveling in every rise, fall, twist and turn.

To every soul who has taken their precious time to read my story and poems, I bow to you now with a message of peace and love from my heart.

Namaste to you all,

Edwina

THOUGHTS
AND FEELINGS

Edwina as always every poem you have done has been inspirational and so heartfelt, and have summed up how all of us warriors have felt at some point. You really deserve this.

Maria Walsh, 48, Surrey

I am so proud of you Edwina! The words in your poems touched me so often and in so many ways. You managed to capture the essence of various feelings and experiences during my TNBC journey. Wishing you love, health and happiness.

Laura Low-Douse, 39, TNBC warrior.

Edwina's poems say everything us fellow cancer sufferers have thought but not been able to put into words to talk with others. They really helped me whilst I was recovering. Although we have never met she is a true inspiration.

Jeanne Hudson

Edwina and I went through treatment for TNBC at the same time. She found her gift for expressing the hopes/fears/worries and highs of this journey (yes there are some highs - and Edwina captures the essence of them in the most perfect way).

Vicky Noble

There are days we have laughed and cried collectively as one of our band of TN warriors gets good news or loses the battle against this awful disease. But through it all Edwina has kept us entertained and expressed how we were all feeling in the most enigmatic way. I have lots of love for this lady.

Vicky, 42, Ramsbottom, TNBC warrior

I love every poem you have written but the one that really hit home was 'Who am I? I love that one line "but it will grow back cheap words in the air". I get choked up still reading that one. I can't wait for the book; fantastic news.

Amanda Jane Luke, Her2 positive, 42, Norton, Stoke on Trent.

I love reading your poems Edwina. There's one for every mood I am feeling! They're raw and realistic of what this journey brings us on. There's respect for the warriors we have lost and warriors who are struggling with secondaries and of course I love our chant! Well done and always excited to read more.

Sarah McSherry, 30, Dublin.

Edwina and Julie were my rocks during chemo, we were the Three Amigos. Sadly Julie didn't make it but she is forever in our hearts. Our friendship means the world to me; Edwina can put down in words exactly how it feels to suffer from TNBC. It's a special gift and something that I can't do. We are still the two amigos and will be friends forever.

Cath, 54, Leigh, Lancashire

I feel quite humble adding to this thread as I'm neither a warrior nor a survivor but cancer took my Dad away from me without any warnings and very quickly and I still struggle each day, but Edwina you are an inspiration and a real ray of light.

Gill Rodden

Your poems have really helped me to get through, Edwina. It's a worrying time going through treatment and to have words of encouragement from someone who's done it inspired me and has shown me I could get through it all too. It's ok doctors and nurses telling us what will happen but you can say it exactly as it is because you've been through it. I personally needed to know it from a survivor to become a survivor too. Thank you from the bottom of my heart.

Sue Belcher, Leicestershire, Ovarian Cancer Survivor

All your poems I've read have been brilliant Edwina. You describe exactly how we feel and what we go through when fighting this horrible disease. I wish you all the best with publishing your book and look forward to buying some for friends and family. Hopefully through your words they can understand how it actually feels. I hid a lot away from them and they only saw me once in a wig and makeup and my smiley face was on. The poem I relate to most is "Who am I?"

**Dianne Hutchison, 55, fellow breast warrior,
Buckie, Scotland**

Edwina, from one of your TNBC Warrior sisters, your words are absolutely from the heart and they touch my soul. They bring tears and laughter and it's as though you know exactly what we ladies have gone and are going through. You are talented, heartfelt and encouraging, keep writing.

Karen Ward

Edwina I have followed your journey from the beginning. I have been so inspired by your poems and they have given me hope and strength. Each poem you have written reflects so many other people's experiences and puts into words how people actually feel and thank you so much for that! I wish you all the success for the publication of your book and I can't wait to have a copy of my own. Thank you from the bottom of my heart.

Judy Stafford

I love all of Edwina's poems; they are inspirational, educational and truly heartfelt. They sum up the myriad of emotions a cancer diagnosis produces.

Gill Ramsden, 53, Halifax.

Well done Edwina, bright blessings to you.

Dawn Whitehouse

That is fantastic! Well done Edwina.

Kelly Bailey

Edwina, you are one big shining star and an example to us all. And hey you are going to become famous with your dogs.

Linda Mair

Well done -you deserve it.

Ruthy Fletcher

Since virtually meeting you through Yoga, we connected because of our BC experience. Your words are the perfect literal antidote to the fear, doubt, panic and dehumanising effects of a cancer diagnosis; and the journey through treatment and it's aftermath. Helping to dispel the myths and exposing the truths of attitudes of others and ourselves. The results bring happiness.

Isabel Brooks

You deserve this Edwina, such an inspiration to all. You are so talented. Love to you well done.

Diane Owen

Your poems are raw, realistic, uplifting, authentic and an inspirational read. I've been moved to tears by some of your work. Not just because my Mother died from breast cancer at the very young age of 42, but also as I have a number of survivor friends who have loved your words too and who echo your braveness. You speak from the heart and soul and have used your yogic approach to highlight the ups and downs of your own personal battle. Truly inspiring and when your book is published it'll be on my list to give out as presents to students, friends and family. I love how your work is not just about the 'cancer' either - it also projects your amazingly resilient attitude to life in general. Thank you for sharing - a true Yogi. Namaste

Mandy Nichols

As you know, 'Hippo Days' has a very special place in my heart.

David Parkes

A FINAL WORD TO YOGIS AND YOGINIS OUT THERE

Ahimsa

I just thought I would add a little kindness advice from my experience of teaching yoga for the last 7 years and from the journey I have found myself on for the last 20 months. This is not just for yoga instructors but for anyone who practises yoga of any sort.

I found yoga during a huge breakdown/traumatic time in my life in June 2010 and it not only saved me but transformed me. In time I got better, left my job and became an instructor myself.

I absolutely loved my job teaching yoga (and still do) and was happy to embrace just about any styles. I had begun with very little flow or Vinyasa in my classes or in my personal practise, preferring Hatha based. But as the years progressed, I found myself drawn to teaching much more dynamic lessons, stronger and faster moving- pushing myself and students further.

Now this was great, my students loved it and I loved it! I took on more classes, my body looked amazing (especially for my age) and I genuinely thought this is it- I can do this into my old age. I'm the fittest (and healthiest) I've ever been! As I got stronger and more flexible, I was able to achieve asanas I couldn't have done as a teenage gymnast. Maybe I let ego get in the way (or the pressures to teach those challenging asana)? We're yoga teachers yes, but we're human too and less than perfect. (No matter how much kale we consume or meditation we do!) Then out of the blue, I developed back pain, crippling back pain. I couldn't even do a cat stretch at times. I went to every therapy going, but never got to the bottom of it back then.

Then breast cancer stopped me in my tracks in January 2017. I knew this was a huge warning sign to stop and not just to slow down! I learnt more about 'yoga' while I battled a rare and cruel type of cancer than I had in thousands of hours of asana/meditation on my mat. Undergoing treatments I had sworn I would never use and seeing my naive perfect little world 'crumble'. I'm telling you this, why? Because we are not invincible- our bodies can only take so much. The more we find ourselves demonstrating, taking on more classes, doing hours on our mat, pushing our bodies and minds to the limit- we become like professional athletes. Yet athletes have long rest and recovery periods and of course they retire younger.... do we? It's not just physical what we do, we are giving of our minds, hearts and souls too. Remember that and be kind to yourself first: that body won't last forever.

An MRI looking for cancer some months back showed up the accelerated degeneration in my body from too much asana; the damage I had actually done to myself. Please, please I implore you, be careful.

So here I am teaching again, but soooo gentle now. My own practise looks nothing like it did and I love it more. I have neuropathy from chemotherapy, joint pain and arthritis from the radiotherapy, and I am in a lot of pain at times. Yet I am happier than I have ever been. I write poetry of course and I write: a thing that has also become my 'yoga' and doesn't need a 'chaturanga' or headstand to do it.

I stop when I need to. I recognise when my body, mind, heart and soul need to make changes again or slow down a bit. Do you? Please, please, please, be kind to yourselves. We are not invincible, perfect or gurus- we are human beings. In the words many of us use so often- 'Ahimsa' non-violence and compassion for all beings. So remember to always begin that wonderful word with you, never forgetting what incredible human beings and souls that you are.

Namaste

ACKNOWLEDGEMENTS

Wow, where do I start when it comes to saying thank you? There are so many people to thank over the last 20 months for helping, supporting and guiding me. I can honestly say, without them all- I wouldn't be as happy and healthy as I am today.

Firstly, my thanks go to my partner, my daughters and my mum. They, above everyone else, have been there on a daily basis. It was they who picked me up at my worst times, who made me laugh when I felt dreadful, who said daily prayers for me, who had an unwavering love and kindness towards me and never once let me down. Then thanks go to my extended family for their constant kindness and support, my sisters and brothers, my nieces and nephews, my cousins and Aunty and Uncle.

Also a special thank you goes to my cousin David Thompson, who has worked through the whole of this book to proof read and offer his encouragement and advice (Missed typos are me!). I have been overwhelmed by his kind words and inspiration to keep going, a true kindred spirit I am honoured to say. This book would not exist without his help- that's for sure!

My thanks go to Julie's family- her husband, children, mum, dad, brother, sister-in-law, nephew, family and friends. They have been an invaluable source of support during the writing of this book and a constant reminder to me of why I was writing. I hope and I pray that Julie's spirit does shine through in my words and that many who never even met her, will feel the love and kindness that radiated from this lady.

Thanks of course also go to Julie herself, my muse. She was the inspiration for so much of my poetry and my blogging. Every word I wrote for her and about her will rest in my heart as long as I shall live. I will continue no doubt to have my 'Hippo

Days', but Julie will be there to remind me of how lucky I am to be alive. So I thank you my friend, for everything.

Many thanks go to my friends. There hasn't been a week gone by, when at least one of them hasn't text me, messaged me or even visited. They have lent kindness, laughter and love to me throughout. Thank you to you all- Lynn, Wendy A, Carol, Cath Q, Sharon, Lis, Angie, Katya, Juliette, Rachael, Wendy P, Paul, Ellen, Callie, Fiona, Hayley (for the haircuts!), Darren, Toby, Jo B, Rachael M and of course to the many friends I have on social media who have sent so many kind words and their endless love.

My thanks go to my students, the 'Warrior Tribe' who rose up around me to offer their help in my hour of need. Christine Sch, Karen, Christine Sh, Anne, Deb, Jayne, Ros, Claire P, Claire K, Alex, Kev, Ashgar, Viv, Shirley, Tim, Juliet, Emma D, Sandra, Lynn T, Stella, Rita, Penny, Gladys, Arthur, Gill, Julie Mc, Jenny K, Audrey, Andrea, Kieran, Holly, Dawn, David, Andy, Karen, Catherine, Anne-Marie, Alan, Faith, Jessie, Nina, Chetna, Joey, Keeley, Maria, Peter, Priya, Maureen, Neil, Charlotte and Rita. My thanks also goes to the many more students (there are too many to name), members, staff and management at DW Leigh, DW Bolton, DW Warrington, DW Trafford, Total Fitness Walkden, Total Fitness Bolton and Lotusfloweryoga studios in Leigh. I especially thank you for the fundraisers that were organised as they were invaluable during my treatments and to my on-going recovery.

My thanks go to the wealth of Yoga Instructors who stepped up to cover my classes, offer their support and in some cases, take over those classes for me. I have been truly grateful for how the Yoga community has held me closely throughout. Wendy A, Julie T, Jane L, Julie N, Pete, Lesley-Anne, Chris A, Karen, Lisa, Louise, Donna, Katya, Sarah D, Will, Adi, Laura B, Isabel, Ellen, Wendy W, Kay, Holly, Adele, Ross, Belinda and Will.

My thanks go to my friends at school past and present, those of whom have been friends and not colleagues for many years. Vannessa, Trish, Nigel, Fr Mc, Janet, Mary, Suzanne, Louise, Maggie, Vicky, Pauline, Magda, Catherine, Laura, Audra, Phil and every one at SSPP who have offered their kinds words of support.

A special thank you must go to the group Triple Negative Warriors UK, Carole Anne, Colista and each and every member in there. I have been blessed to meet many of these ladies and am grateful for their unwavering love, advice and encouragement throughout my journey. It is from them that I am often inspired to write. There are so many ladies who have been especially supportive, so my thanks go to you all. In particular, thank you to Cath, Jo and Debbie for the many times we've managed to meet up too! A huge thank you goes especially to those ladies who allowed me to add their poems and also to Emma Knowles for the use of her brilliant TN blog. Thank you to so many of you who provided me with the sunflower pictures, they were all stunning and a special thank you to Melonie Wallace for allowing me to use her image.

A huge thank you goes to the many contributors who funded the publishing of my book- without you it simply wouldn't exist! Wendy Brooks, Katerina G, Danille M, Nigel C, Susan D, Chris P, Shirley P, Louise R, Dianne H, Emma C, Andy A and Rosemary C.

My thanks go to the many people who have been following my poems and blogs on social media. You have encouraged my creativity every step of the way and I truly hope that this book will live up to your expectations.

My thanks also to Breast Cancer Care for allowing me to use their picture in the poem 'A Heart On A Wall' and to Fiona Law for the mention of her Yoga Nidra 'Fertile Darkness'.

Also, of course, a huge thank you goes to The Shine Bright Foundation and Jacky Atkinson for their wonderful work towards a cure for Triple Negative breast cancer. I thank them for their foreword in this book, but especially for the work and fund raising they have achieved in such a few short years. It is thanks to them that trials are now taking place at Christies to find a more effective treatment for TN. Maybe even one day, they will be instrumental in finding a cure.

Finally my thanks of course go to the NHS- the nurses, doctors, oncologists, surgeons, receptionists, staff and volunteers who are there to help and support you every step of the way. I thank all of those at The Christie in Wigan, the Thomas Linacre Centre, Leigh Infirmary, Salford Royal and the Royal Albert Hospital in Wigan. Your dedication to the health and healing of complete strangers is inspirational.

I genuinely pray there is no one I have left out. I have had so much support, kindness, love and a wealth of cards, flowers and gifts. Each and every single thing I have received has been treasured, be it love or the simplest of gestures. I thank each and everyone one of you, you have been my inspiration, my encouragement and my healing force.

Namaste

Edwina

INDEX OF POEMS

INDEX OF BLOGS

Lightning Source UK Ltd.
Milton Keynes UK
UKHW051950271118
333078UK00009B/227/P